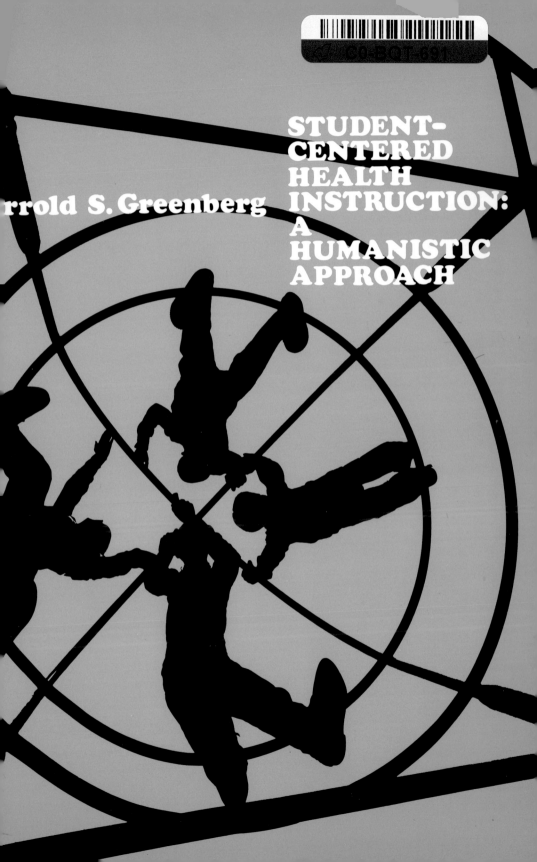

STUDENT-
CENTERED
HEALTH
INSTRUCTION:
A
HUMANISTIC
APPROACH

rrold S. Greenberg

STUDENT-CENTERED HEALTH INSTRUCTION

A Humanistic Approach

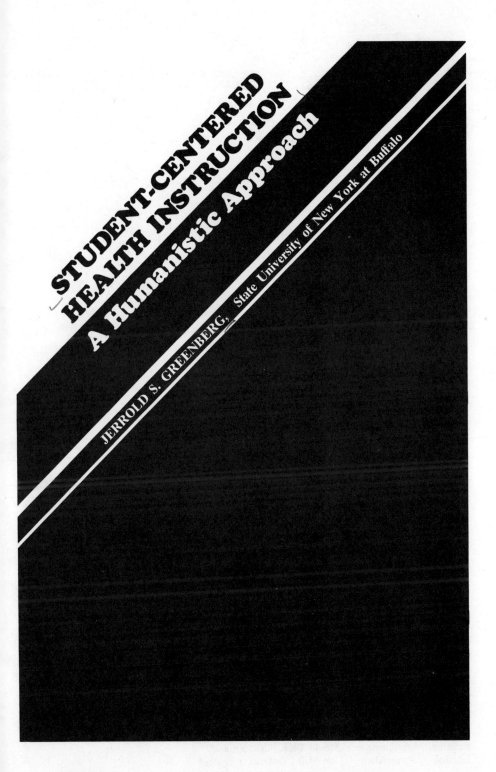

STUDENT-CENTERED HEALTH INSTRUCTION

A Humanistic Approach

JERROLD S. GREENBERG, State University of New York at Buffalo

For the in-class photographs in this book, the author is grateful to:

Zennon Detutat and
Payne Junior High School
North Tonowanda, N. Y.

Patricia Marcklinger and
Amherst Central Senior High School
Amherst, N. Y.

ADDISON-WESLEY PUBLISHING COMPANY
Reading, Massachusetts • Menlo Park, California
London • Amsterdam • Don Mills, Ontario • Sydney

I thank you so much,
Karen my wife,
For typing and reading
And bearing my strife.

To Todd, my son,
I only can say,
I'll make up the time
we missed out on play.

To Keri, my girl,
as you will grow,
I hope this book
will love help you know.

To all of my students
and friends there at school,
I'll always remember
your bearing this fool.

And lastly, but surely,
To Mom and to Dad,
much of you is in
this very proud lad.

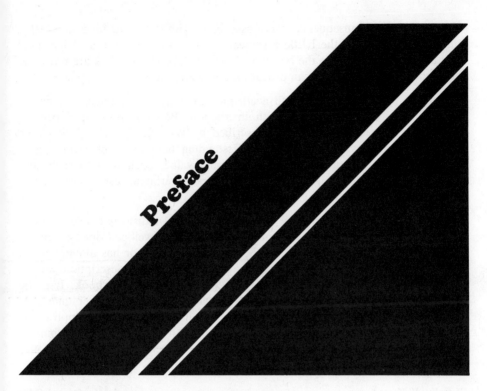

Preface

Have you ever thought how much school is like war?
Classes like battles?
Free periods like truces?
Teachers' lounges and student cafeteria like military camps?

Both sides seem committed to battling for 40 or so minutes, resting, and then resuming battle. During the confrontation teachers utilize weapons such as grading, motivation, hand raising, and parental visitations; whereas students employ calling out, passing notes, trips to the lavatory, truancy, and daydreaming.

At long last the class period ends and the teacher retreats to lick his or her wounds. The retreat invariably ends in the teachers' lounge where new strategies are conceived. First a cup of coffee to stimulate the body; next, conversation with fellow soldiers to benefit from their experiences; and lastly, the formulation of new or revised strategies to be employed when the battle resumes. With a pat on the back from compatriots indicative of their unwavering support, the teacher leaves the safety afforded by the camp and once again enters the field of battle.

What is the "other side" doing during the truce? The students often retreat to the school cafeteria where they too lick their wounds. First a hamburger, coke, and french fries (with plenty of ketchup on all but the coke); next, conversation with fellow soldiers to learn of their reactions to strategies employed by opposing soldiers and what consequences were associated with such reactions; and lastly, plans for action when the battle resumes are agreed upon. With a "Right on," the students, upon hearing the bell indicating the opposing soldiers are refreshed and ready to go, leave their camp bent on not losing the war.

Although a tragic situation for all academic disciplines, the antagonistic nature of schooling spells doom for health instruction. Perhaps more appropriately designated "education for life," as described by Whitehead,* health education requires mutual trust, respect, and understanding between teacher and pupil. Without teacher-student rapport, attitudes and values pertaining to such controversial topics as premarital sexual intercourse, marijuana use, abortion, and mental health will seldom be expressed.

What follows will undoubtedly be criticized by some as a distorted view of health instruction. Through myopic eyes and a biased heart, developed during years of teaching children and young adults about health, the author has attempted (in Chapter 1) to describe health instruction as it is today. The description, admittedly, is subjective because subjectivity is characteristic of this book. It is the desire of the author for health educators to relate to students rather than content; to be less objective and more subjective. If, in attempting to accomplish this task, the author has exaggerated and elaborated to an extent that is disturbing to the reader, forgiveness is sought by way of subsequent chapters which offer means for developing more relevant health education.

Buffalo, N.Y.   J.S.G.
July 1977

---

* Alfred North Whitehead, *The Aims of Education And Other Essays* (New York: The Macmillan Company, 1929).

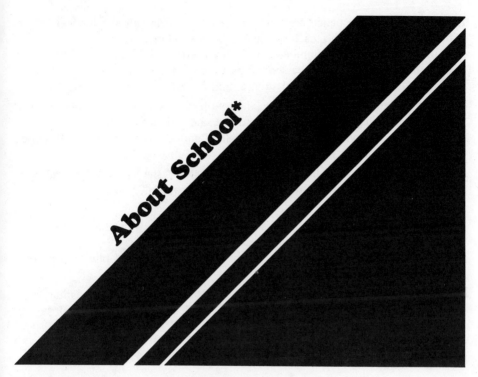

About School*

He always wanted to say things. But no one understood.
He always wanted to explain things. But no one cared.
So he drew.

Sometimes he would just draw and it wasn't anything. He wanted to carve it in
stone or write it in the sky.
He would lie out on the grass and look up in the sky, and it would be only him
and the sky and the things inside him that needed saying.
And it was after that, that he drew the picture. It was a beautiful picture. He
kept it under the pillow and would let no one see it.
And he would look at it every night and think about it. And when it was dark,
and his eyes were closed, he could still see it.
And it was all of him. And he loved it.

When he started school, he brought it with him. Not to show anyone, but just to
have it with him like a friend.

It was funny about school.
He sat in a square, brown desk like all the other square, brown desks and he
thought it should be red.
And his room was a square, brown room. Like all the other rooms. And it was
tight and close. And stiff.

* Source unknown.

He hated to hold the pencil and the chalk, with his arm still and his feet flat on the floor, stiff, with the teacher watching and watching.

And then he had to write numbers. And they weren't anything. They were worse than the letters that could be something if you put them together.

And the numbers were tight and square, and he hated the whole thing.

The teacher came and spoke to him. She told him to wear a tie like all the other boys. He said he didn't like them, and she said it didn't matter.

After that they drew. And he drew all yellow and it was the way he felt about morning. And it was beautiful.

The teacher came and smiled at him. "What's this?" she said. "Why don't you draw something like Ken's drawing? Isn't that beautiful?"

It was all questions.

After that his mother bought him a tie, and he always drew airplanes and rocket ships like everyone else. And he threw the old picture away.

And when he lay out alone looking at the sky, it was big and blue and all of everything, but *he* wasn't anymore.

He was square inside and brown, and his hands were stiff, and he was like anyone else. And the thing inside him that needed saying didn't need saying anymore.

It had stopped pushing. It was crushed. Stiff.

Like everything else.

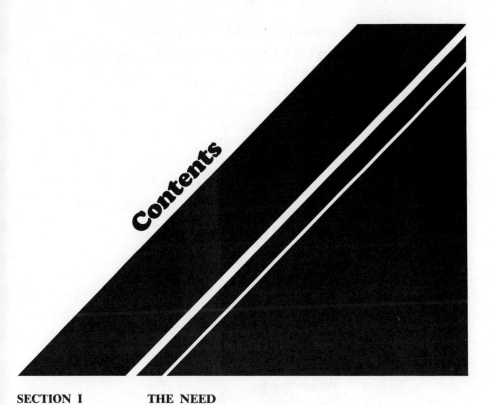

Contents

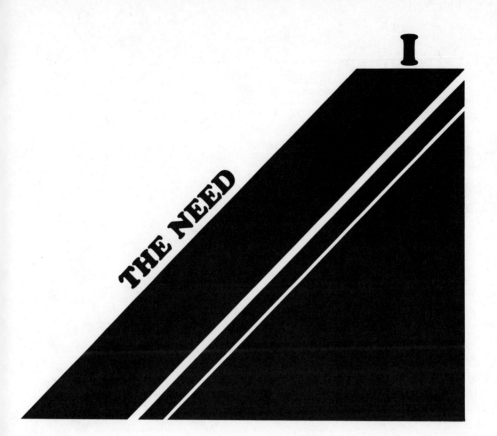

THE NEED

I

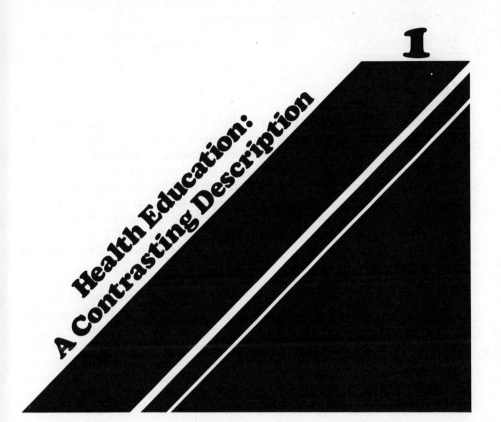

1

Health Education: A Contrasting Description

A t first glance, attempting to describe health instruction would seem to be a formidable task. One may assume the myriad of health education curricula offered would contraindicate generalizations pertaining to health education. It is readily admitted there will be exceptions to the pictures painted below; and in fact there are communities boasting health education curricula presently in revision. However, far too many health instructional programs can be stereotyped, and the stereotype is not flattering. In the face of this realization, though, some excellent health education programs call to be recognized. The differences in these programs encompass the functions and roles of teachers and students, and the courses themselves.

This chapter is an attempt to describe the two extremes on the continuum of health education programs—the rigid, highly structured type, and the flexible, informal type. The author's bias toward the latter will be obvious and explained throughout. There will be no panacea offered for all the woes which are bemoaned. However, before a journey is completed a first step must be taken. The reader is asked to slip into his or her pedagogical shoes and tread, with the author, down the path of concern. Though it is a threatening journey—change tends to be threatening—the rewards are more than satisfactory. Subsequent journeys of a similar nature will be anticipated with exultation. For you see, once a pedagogical journeyman, always a pedagogical journeyman. With an aim at accuracy, and an apology for passion, these descriptions begin.

THE HEALTH EDUCATION COURSE

Objectives

In some schools children are expected to attend, be pleasant, be malleable, and learn what they are told to learn. Some health instruction provides no exception to this analysis. Within this type of health instruction, health educators predetermine the objectives for the health instructional experience and term those objectives "health." By way of example, children are taught to appreciate community health agencies. When later they find a discrepancy in quality and quantity of health care for whites and nonwhites,[1,2] they and we are perplexed. One need only scan health education curricula to acquire evidence indicating predetermined education objectives and lack of student involvement in the planning of these objectives.

Aside from nondemocratic procedures pertaining to the formulation of health instructional objectives, the objectives are poorly stated. An objective worded "To understand the harmful effects of drug abuse," cannot be accurately evaluated. One may question the meaning of the word "understand." How can one measure understanding? Can one measure states of mind? One may question the term "harmful effects." What effects? Physiological? Sociological? Legal? In addition *one would need more information* pertaining to the term "drug abuse." It becomes readily apparent upon screening health education programs that, in some cases, the objectives, if stated, cannot be evaluated in a valid and reliable manner.[3] In summary, some health instruction courses tend to be based upon objectives which are neither democratically selected nor capable of being measured.

"If you are teaching skills that cannot be evaluated, you are in the awkward position of being unable to demonstrate that you are teaching anything at all."[4] So writes one of the more noteworthy proponents of behavioral objectives (sometimes referred to as performance objectives, operational objectives, or instructional objectives). Mager suggests that objectives be stated in a manner which provides for an evaluation of their achievement. Three criteria are cited by Mager to guide the reader in stating objectives behaviorally. They are:

a. Identify the terminal behavior; i.e., what the learner will be expected to do at the end of the learning experience.
b. Describe the important conditions under which the behavior will be expected to occur.
c. Specify the criteria of acceptable performance; i.e., how well the learner must perform to be acceptable.[5]

An example of a health instructional objective of which Mager might be expected to approve is:

Given selected hereditary characteristics of two people, the student can apply the principle of dominant-recessive heredity characteristics to a prediction of possible inherited characteristics of the couple's offspring.[6]

If stated more generally, such an objective might be impossible to adequately evaluate.

In this objective the terminal behavior is to "apply the principle of dominant-recessive hereditary characteristics . . . ," the important condition is "given selected hereditary characteristics of two people . . . ," and the criteria of acceptable performance is implied in that the principle of dominant-recessive hereditary characteristics should be applied with total accuracy and consistent with the laws of heredity proposed by Mendel.

The limiting considerations of lack of training in stating objectives behaviorally and lack of time in which to mull over objectives have led to the establishment of the Instructional Objectives Exchange (IOX). The Exchange serves as a clearinghouse for behavioral objectives and, for a nominal fee, will mail to interested persons objectives submitted by educators throughout the country. Though still in the developmental stages, IOX possesses materials which may be helpful to the health educator.[7]

The use of behavioral objectives in health instruction serves several purposes. Of importance appears to be the possibility of objectively evaluating the health instructional experience. Often required to justify their very existence, some health educators have little data to support their position. However, if objectives are stated behaviorally, their achievement can easily be documented. On the other hand, if it was determined that the health instructional objectives were not successfully accomplished, appropriate adjustments in the learning experience might be indicated. The realization of the need for changes in the program, and the subsequent making of those changes, could result in a health education program of which school personnel, students, and parents could be proud.

Another advantage of the behavioral objective approach seems to be the necessity for clarifying the purposes of the health instructional program. When stating health instruction objectives behaviorally, the teacher must be concerned, for instance, with whether the objective is for the student to have knowledge pertaining to drugs or for the student not to abuse drugs. Once health instructional objectives are clarified, content selection and learning experiences can be more adequately chosen. One of the objections to the use of behavioral objectives pertains to the lack of student involvement and its nondemocratic nature. These shortcomings, however, need not be typical. Although some teachers might predetermine objectives and appear to "program" students to satisfy such objectives, as a computer might be programmed, other teachers might work with students to arrive at a mutual statement of objectives for the class. The following questions are offered by way of example and may be helpful in allowing students to clarify their own objectives:

a. What do we want to know about the environment?
b. How many different areas of environmental health do we want to investigate? What are they? How should we proceed?
c. Do we just want to study the environment or do we want to do something about it?

Such a sequence of questions would guide students and teachers in determining what content will be investigated, how information will be obtained, and what action will be taken at the end of the learning experience. The effect of this procedure is analyzed elsewhere in this chapter. Suffice it to say that students will thereby assume greater responsibility for their learning than is presently the case, since they will determine for themselves *what* they will learn, *how* they will learn it, and how they will *apply* their learning.

Simply because an objective is stated behaviorally does not, however, necessarily imply that such an objective is an appropriate one. While objectives in health education must be perceived as meaningful by the pupils involved, and of course be educationally sound, they must also be decided upon after several variables are considered. What is possible financially in one school may not be possible in another. In addition, instructional time, community resources, and administrative support should not be overlooked. The reader can probably cite other factors which limit what can be accomplished through health instruction. The health instructor, however, must guard against the use of rationalization to explain away a shoddy health education program. Much can be done with what is available. The hope for meaningful health instruction relates to a change in roles of teachers and students rather than more equipment, facilities, or community resources. With a realistic approach to the limitations of the health instructional experience, students and teachers alike can determine valid objectives for the program.

Content

The content investigated in some health education classes is often categorized into packages. Examples of packages, pedagogically referred to as units, are consumer health education, drug education, sex education, nutrition education, and alcohol education. Very often packages are chosen before the formulation of objectives. By way of example, the inclusion of drug education in the school curriculum has been a reaction to drug abuse in the community. School personnel chose the package of drug education and then proceeded to debate the objectives desired from the ingestion of the package's contents. Should drug education be directed at preventing the behavior referred to as drug abuse? or should it be informational, thereby allowing for variant decisions related to drug behavior which, when incorporated within differing value structures, become rational?

As do procedures for the determination of health education objectives, content selection incorporates little student involvement in some health education programs. Students are not allowed to select packages from the supermarket shelves but rather are given a shopping bag which includes packages selected by the management. Like a homemaker, the student who is not satisfied with the bag's contents might be heard to complain, "But I've had cornflakes, know about cornflakes, and don't want any more cornflakes!"

In other health programs, students are involved in content selection. That educators perched upon a pedestal decide the content of Johnny's health program without asking Johnny what he's interested in or what he needs seems to be the height of absurdity. Rather than inflexible predetermination of content offerings (e.g., bicycle safety will be studied in the sixth grade, while abortion will be discussed in the twelfth grade), it appears reasonable to assume that topics students discuss out of class (perhaps on the street corner) should be appropriate topics for discussion within class. The vast variance in child development indicates a need for individualization in content offerings to the extent that each child can investigate those areas to which his or her life, at that moment, has led him or her to perceive a need or interest. It must be apparent that this type of education requires roles dissimilar to those presently adopted by students and faculty. A further discussion of educational role changes is offered in another section of this chapter. It seems necessary to add that methodology to elicit concerns of students relative to content is available. The fishbowl technique, described elsewhere in this book, is one method which can be employed for this purpose.

In summary, all content is fair game for the classroom, with a *desire to know* the criterion by which content is selected.

The Required Course

In many school districts, enrollment in a health education course is a prerequisite for graduation.[8] Health educators seem to be in favor of such a requirement and cite what appear to be valid considerations to support this position:

a. Status of health education and health instructors would be enhanced by ascribing such importance to the discipline that courses are required.

b. Skills and knowledge taught in health education classes are of such a nature that everyone must possess these skills and knowledge to live a healthy life.

c. With subject areas competing for limited school finances, health education may very well be overlooked. If health education were a requirement, finance would of necessity be provided.

It would be inaccurate to relay the impression that health education is a required course in all schools. Many school districts provide health instruction to those who identify an interest in that area, while other school districts do not offer health instruction at all.

It is wise to remember, though, that within every required course of study many electives are possible. For example, a required drug education class may be able to elect which drugs to study, means of study (independent study, group discussion, field trips), and methods of evaluation. However, required courses are anathema to the type of health instruction advocated in this book. As students should be able to select objectives and content for health instructional experiences, they should likewise be able to select, or not to select, these experiences in the first place. In this manner, health educators will be required to develop health education course offerings which will be meaningful to, and viewed as meaningful by, the students. The pupils will be transformed into buyers in an open market. If it is worth the price—a time commitment—health instruction will be bought; if not worth the price, health instruction will not be selected. Responsiveness to students' needs and interests would then, if health instructors intended to maintain their employment status, be necessitated. Some health education programs are presently operating, and thriving, on just such a free-market basis.

The Noncredit Course

The arguments offered for awarding "credit" for health instruction are similar to those related to requiring enrollment in health instruction by all students.

An additional consideration is said to be the attitude of students toward the health instructional experience. It is suggested that students will view health education as more valuable, and thereby manifest behaviors more conducive to learning, if credit is awarded. As with required health education, practices pertaining to alloting credit for health education are varied.

The concerns of health educators regarding the awarding of credit for health instructional experiences relate to their desire for increased status of health education and greater student motivation. However, if students are allowed to elect health instruction, if once enrolled they can choose content and learning experiences, and if the course of study is made responsive to student needs and interests, then health education will be spoken of in positive terms and student motivation for learning about health will be vastly increased. Therefore, in view of the type of health instruction being advocated in this chapter, a discussion of the merits or demerits of awarding credit for health education classes appears to be irrelevant.

Classroom Facility

There is a tendency for schools alternating health instruction with physical education to meet in any available space. Expediency being a consideration, classrooms chosen often are close to the gymnasium. The author has visited one school where health instruction was conducted in a small gymnasium. The pupils sat on the floor, chairs and desks were not available, and the teacher stood in the middle of the gymnasium. While this example may be an exception, there are many schools which utilize inappropriate settings for health instructional experiences. Other schools provide classrooms equipped with ample space, adequate lighting and appropriate ventilation; some are even equipped with portable chairs and desks. However, conducive settings for health instruction tend to be positively correlated with a scheduling practice of separate or correlated health education courses of study.

Enactive vs. Reactive

A professor in whose class this author was fortunate to be a student once remarked, "Education tends to be reactive rather than enactive." This statement can be appropriately directed toward some health instruction. As previously stated, drug education has been a reaction to drug abuse in the community. Environmental health education has been a reaction to a societal problem. Sex education has been a reaction to what has been termed a "sexual revolution." One can only wonder how many people would presently be drug addicts if drug education had been enacted, how many rivers would be polluted if environmental health programs had been enacted, and what the incidence of venereal disease might be if sex education had been enacted. Topics such as ethical and moral considerations of genetic manipulation and implantation of body organs will only be debated in some schools when a reaction to an already evidenced problem is required; whereas such a debate is raging presently in the better health education courses of study.

K-12 Curriculum

If health instruction is to become a meaningful experience for students which will allow them to investigate topics with which they are concerned, each student must have an opportunity to enroll in health education classes each semester of his or her schooling. To insist that interests in health topics be channeled into specific semesters is to insist that interests will not be satisfied when learning will be most meaningful and retention of learning therefore most to be expected. What is then suggested is not a K-12 curriculum in health instruction as presently conceived by educators, but rather a K-12 curriculum in health instruction which will be placed upon the shelf of educational offerings and always available to, but not required of, the student. By use of varied methods of instruction and learning aids, and in view of the changing role of the instructor, the health teacher need not be overly concerned with the K-12 curriculum herein conceived resulting in densely populated classes or in sparse enrollments. Both sized classes may be offered meaningful health educational experiences.

The scheduling problems associated with such an educational approach are not as difficult as first perceived. Past experience in scheduling similar courses, surveys of students' interests, and subjective assessments by students of teachers' effectiveness can help in predicting which offerings students will subscribe to in large numbers. Such offerings can be established as large group sessions. Other experiences of a more specific nature, to which sparse student enrollment is anticipated, can be scheduled as independent study projects supervised by the health instructor. Perhaps a more exotic manner of scheduling experiences for only a handful of students would be to establish areas within the school library, or another classroom, which are equipped with cassette tape recorders, filmstrip projectors, film previewers, programmed texts, etc. for students' use. The software employed with this equipment can be stored by the instructor for distribution when appropriate to students' objectives.

THE STUDENT

Economically, education has been viewed as either a consumptive good or an investment good. It's been suggested that people consume education just as they eat hamburgers and attend the cinema, or they are future-oriented and are willing to be educated for gains accruing upon completion of the educational process.[9] There seems to be a third possibility associated with compulsory education; i.e., students who are neither consuming nor investing but have no choice other than to be in attendance. Some health educators advocating health instruction as a required course of study would compel students, originally compelled to attend school, to attend health instructional classes. The consequences of the realization of this aim are evident in the motivation, attitude, and behavior of students, as well as their retention of learning related to health education. Other health educators philosophically opposed to such requirements, it seems to this author, have a different experience. Increased motivation for learning of health concepts, better attitude toward health instruction and health instructors, and a greater potential for the retention of health learning appear to be the more profound concomitants of student-centered health instruction.

Motivation

It would appear to be a difficult task to conduct a conversation or activity with youngsters upon which sex or drugs were the principal foci and have that conversation or activity be uninteresting. Yet some health education instructors seem equal to such a task. This author has witnessed a discussion pertaining to premarital sexual intercourse conducted in such a manner as to elicit such extraneous activities on the part of students as:

a. The completion of a crossword puzzle.
b. The reading of the sports page of a local newspaper.
c. The agreement on plans for an after-school activity.

True, not all health education classes are so conducted. However, a number can be so categorized.

Evidence of students' motivations regarding attendance of some health instructional classes can be readily observed. Witness the facial expressions and movement patterns of students upon entering the health education classroom. They may show lethargy and hesitancy to commence the class' activities, as well as smirks and shrugs when the teacher asks for the students' attention. By way of contrast, the author has visited a health education class where the learning process was begun by the students before the teacher was in attendance. Upon the teacher's arrival, a chair was provided and the discussion continued. Unfortunately, such learning experiences tend to be the exception rather than the rule.[10]

Presently, regarding student motivation related to the learning of health concepts, the question health educators often ask of themselves is: "How can I *make them* want to learn what *I* want to teach them?" Health educators utilizing the student-centered approach to health instruction transform this question into: "How can I *help them* learn what *they* want to learn?" It is obvious the focus is thus shifted from the teacher to the students. The students, previously receptors of knowledge presented by the teacher, now become consumers of knowledge they have uncovered. If, as is often proclaimed, teachers do not know a subject until they teach that subject, and an analogy is made between teachers and student, perhaps a student best knows a subject when partly re-

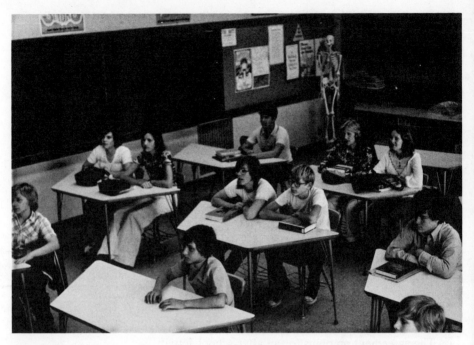

Students seated in traditional ways and who are inactive tend to be difficult to motivate.

sponsible for teaching that subject. If accepted, this statement indicates that not only do students learn best *from* other students, but students learn best when *teaching* other students. If they are allowed to pursue interests in health instruction and assume a large measure of responsibility for their own learning and that of their peers, motivational levels will skyrocket. Such has been the case in Monticello, New York.[11] In student-centered health education classes, the students' intent countenances, raised voices, eager entry into the classroom, and plans for study after school attest to high-level motivation toward health learnings.

Attitude and Behavior

The attitudes of students, often negative toward both school and health instruction, are manifested in ways other than those already described. There are students who react passively to health instruction. Though in attendance, such students are psychological dropouts. They may read newspapers, talk with classmates, or complete homework for other classes. However, the major portion of passive students will appear to be listening and may even nod in agreement periodically. They exhibit the well known "academic stare." When called upon by the teacher, the passive student may be heard to reply, "Would you repeat the question?"

More negatively involved than the passive student is the rebellious one. Not content to "play the game," the rebellious student is constantly challenging the teacher in an attempt to thwart the boredom he or she is experiencing. Indicative of the rebellious student are the following reactions:

a. Absence from class and/or school.
b. Comments such as, "How do you know that, teach?"
c. Bragging about experiences of an antisocial nature.
d. General undisciplined behavior.

The rebellious students tend to be more honest than the passive ones in that they outwardly express their attitudes toward the health instructional process. Though not appreciated for this trait, they are recognized as not having achieved the objectives of the learning experience. Concerned teachers may therefore, for their own sanity as well as the student's welfare, relate learning experiences to the life of the rebellious student. By this perspective, the passive student, due to his or her passivity, may be receiving inferior instruction and a significantly smaller time commitment from the teacher than is the rebellious student.

In most classes there emerges a third type of student. Referred to as "good kids," these students are actively involved in the learning process. They ask questions, offer information, and solicit other students' responses related to the topic being studied. That these students will learn in spite of the teacher's behavior is apparent. Actively involved students can function effectively as part of varied learning processes. Therefore, as with passive students, the learning activities provided by the teacher may not be directed specifically toward the actively involved student.

In schools where health education is viewed as relevant, wanted, and needed, classroom behavior problems are diminished. Topics which are discussed outside of the classroom may now be discussed within it. These topics assume added significance. Drug education or nutrition education no longer are dry academic areas of study, but become exciting areas requiring action on the part of the student. The student who seeks to diet is now allowed to investigate numerous diets and choose one for him- or herself—not when the teacher says to study nutrition but when he or she decides to diet. Students whose friends smoke marijuana can decide to investigate aspects of that drug *when* they are required to arrive at a decision about its use or nonuse—not when the teacher *suspects* they will be required to arrive at that decision.

The attitude of the student becomes positive related to health instruction, the instruction assumes added meaning, and learning experiences are more effective in the achievement of health instructional objectives when student involvement is sought.

Retention of Learning

In view of some health instruction courses, and some motivations, attitudes, and behavior of students, it is no surprise that some students do not learn much of worth related to health. Incidental learning does occur, but is of questionable worth. For example, when the teacher remarks, "You'd better pay attention because this question is just likely to come up on the test," the student learns that his or her responsibility in that class is to guess what is in the teacher's mind.[12] When the teacher comments, "I never took a drink of liquor in my life!" the student learns that teachers are "square."

The small amount of knowledge that is acquired in some health education courses is not long retained. One need only converse with students who have been enrolled in such health education classes to be convinced of the short span of time learnings remain with the student. Obviously, if health education is to result in healthier people, those who have been instructed about health must retain the knowledge necessary for behaving in a healthy manner. The severity of our society's problems and data related to hospital admissions attest to the unhealthy behavior of Americans, thereby lending credence to the premise that there is little significant retention of learning in many health instructional programs.

On the other hand, since topics studied in some student-centered health education classrooms tend to be of immediate concern to students enrolled in such classes, these topics are often associated with behavior. One student studying nutrition will be dieting; another investigating marijuana will be deciding how to behave in relation to that drug. Since behavior is the result of the learning experience, the knowledge obtained and the attitudes acquired are reinforced. If the knowledge is accurate, the results of the behavior may be predicted. If the results are then forthcoming when the behavior is manifested, the knowledge is positively reinforced; if the expected results of the behavior are not observed, the knowledge may be rejected or revised. Similar procedures accompany attitude development. The immediacy of the utilization of the knowledge obtained and attitudes developed, it is suspected, results in greater retention of learning than in nonstudent-centered health instructional programs.

THE TEACHER

The health education teacher is often a transplant from some other discipline. An investigation into the status of health instruction in the Michigan public schools indicated approximately 50 percent of those teaching health had majored in physical education during their undergraduate education; while only 35 percent had minored in health education at the undergraduate level and less than 50 percent majored in health in graduate schools.[13] An awareness of drug abuse and environmental "halitosis" have created teaching positions for health educators that were not previously available. As a reaction to expanded public school

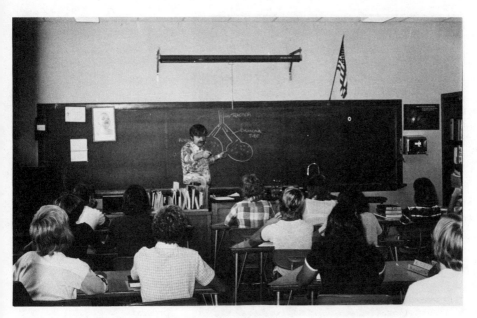

A typical traditional health class in which the teacher is active but the students are passive.

health instructional offerings, colleges and universities are developing increasing numbers of health education teacher preparation programs.[14] It seems safe to assume that future health instructors will be better prepared than are the health teachers of today. Presently, however, a lack of expertise in health education might concern the health teacher and create an attitude of defensiveness. As might be expected, a teacher short of knowledge feels threatened by inquisitive students. Therefore, a nonstimulating atmosphere may be required in such a health education classroom, resulting in the teacher experiencing a sense of frustration.

The Frustrated Teacher

A lack of familiarity with health knowledge is just one factor contributing to a generalized sense of frustration on the part of many health instructors. Another contributing factor is the attitude of students toward health instruction. As previously substantiated, some health education programs are not highly valued by students. Only a uniquely unperceptive teacher remains unaware when students hold health education in low esteem. Low status in students' eyes might be tolerable if other teachers and/or the school administration appreciate the contributions of the health educator. However, health education tends to be viewed as a "frill" in many school curricula, if it is included at all. Since a basic drive of

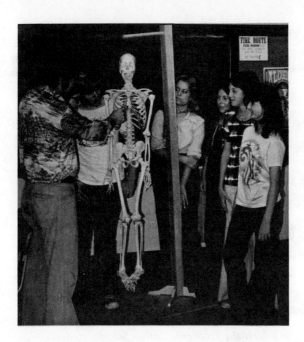

A teacher doesn't have to be a disciplinarian when students are interested and actively involved in the instructional process.

man is toward recognition, the health educator, thwarted in his or her search for professional recognition, may develop a sense of frustration. The practices of scheduling health education after other classes have been scheduled, assigning classrooms for health instruction after other classes have been situated, and providing finances for health instructional aids and equipment after other classes have been apportioned such, do not help to alleviate the self-deprecation characteristic of some health educators.

The Disciplinarian

The classroom behavior of the health instructor may be viewed in relation to the subject matter or the students. Regarding content, some teachers feel a need to infest the classroom with sufficient knowledge to render the students immune from choices of behavior considered unhealthy. However, consistent with the subjective concerns of this book, the teacher's reactions to the students appear to be more informative. As suggested earlier in this chapter, the health instructor interacts with passive, rebellious, and actively involved students. As previously stated, the actively involved student presents little challenge to the teacher, thereby eliciting little in the way of strategies from the teacher that are directed specifically toward the actively involved. The passive student, while of some concern to the teacher, requires only minor responses on the part of the health instructor. Other than requesting the student's attention, a cessation of note passing, and similar administrative responses, the teacher tends to overlook the passive student. The rebellious student, however, does create sufficient anxiety and consternation on the part of the instructor as to require planned strategies. Some health educators, in order to proceed with what may too often appear to be their major concern—content considerations—require obedience and order from all students. Since the rebellious student presents the greatest threat to the type of atmosphere viewed by the teacher as conducive to learning, the teacher is directed in the classroom by thoughts of controlling this student. In effect, the teacher's actions tend to be punitive in nature, the effectiveness of these actions is diminished, and this requires further reactions from the teacher.[15] So, reluctantly, the teacher is reinforcing his or her role as disciplinarian—a role for which he or she has been neither trained nor psychologically prepared.

By way of contrast, some health educators believe that the role of the health instructor as expositor of information is no longer appropriate. Student-centered health instruction maintains a different conception of the teacher. It is assumed that students allowed to pursue interests of their own choosing will choose numerous topics to investigate. To expect the health educator to be knowledgeable in all areas of health is naive at best and dishonest at worst. What, then, is the role played by the health instructors in student-centered health education programs?

The Process Leader

To increase options for students, the health educator must be trained. Training pertaining to the process of learning and group interactions seems most needed. The teacher, no longer filling empty heads with his or her brain's stores, is able to help students achieve their objectives. Since students are expected to interact with fellow students during the learning process, such interaction should be effective. With a knowledge of group dynamics and the means to utilize groups in problem-solving situations, some health educators contribute significantly to the achievement of their students' health instructional objectives. The development of effective leadership, followership, group structure, communication and decision-making are but examples of process concerns which some health educators help students to develop. The acquisition of library skills and the stating of educational objectives behaviorally are additional process concerns to which the teacher's attention is directed.

The Content Consultant

Though recognized as not possessing expertise in all areas of teaching or health, the health instructor does possess knowledge which should be available to students. Upon deciding to investigate community health resources, students may want to avail themselves of the health teacher's knowledge of health agencies. Rather like an annotated bibliography, the health instructor should offer his or her perceptions of the functions and values of numerous agencies. Students may

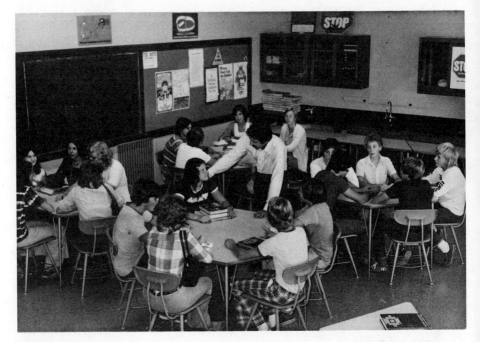

Small-group work is a good means of involving the student in the instructional process.

then decide which agencies to visit, what to look for, and in which order to schedule visitations based on their own desires and additional informational input acquired from the health instructor.

That health teachers do have areas of expertise, however, should not be overlooked. Upon student request, health educators often offer knowledge to students by way of mini-lecture, lecture, or discussion. Additionally, the health educator often provides others who are knowledgeable in specific areas of concern to the class. Areas in which the health instructor can be of help regarding content should be delineated at the outset of the learning experience to the students so they may profit, if so desired, from the teacher as a resource. In essence, the teacher is available to help the students, in whatever way possible, to achieve their objectives in many student-centered health education programs.

As Perceived By Others

The actual value of health instruction for students may be debated. However, a conclusion regarding the worth of health education is relevant only in terms of its effects upon the perceptions of others. People tend to behave in accord with their perceptions of reality; not reality per se. A very tame tiger wandering the streets of New York City will elicit panic reactions from passersby based upon their conception of tigers and their perceptions of that situation. Similarly, students, teachers, and educational administrators, possessing preconceived notions of health education and the health educator, behave in accordance with these notions. Students viewing the health educator as a disciplinarian, the subject matter as irrelevant, and the course of study as being forced upon them, cannot be expected to behave in a manner which learning theorists consider necessary for learning to occur. Consequently, little learning pertaining to health is achieved under those circumstances. Other subject area specialists competing with health educators for the students' time, inheriting students from boring health education classes, and bearing equivalent responsibility for the education of pupils in that school, cannot be viewed as friends of health education or health instructors. And likewise, some school administrators who bear the brunt of parental complaints and aspirations regarding their sons' and daughters' educations, who have previously been students themselves, and who must be concerned with financial implications of school programs, tend to envision health education as a "special" subject.[16] Not to be lost is the effect of the health educator's realization of the aforementioned. Realizing the value ascribed to health instruction by school personnel, the health instructor is none too pleased.

In other school districts the situation is different. The adoption of a new role by the health instructor, one envisioning the teacher as a well to be tapped upon student thirst, results in a new image for health instruction and health instructors. Seen as a help rather than a hindrance, the teacher of health is incorporated into the educational curriculum. As a contributor to the education of students, rather than a determiner of that education, the health educator is welcomed into the students' developmental worlds. When perceived positively by students, other school personnel similarly respond to the health instructor. Parents find their children valuing health instruction, teachers appreciate the change in student attitude and behavior, and school administrators begin hearing of health instruction in a new context—one of satisfaction and enjoyment. An elevating spiral of status, respect, and understanding for health instruction results in a larger portion of the financial pie being apportioned to the health education area, thereby eliminating those limitations placed upon the health program by lack of funds. More funds, more possibilities, better programs, further increased status, etc. The spiral continues upward with decreasing health problems of the school age population in sight.

A WORD ABOUT PARENTS

The emphasis upon the need of a college education is unfortunate. Since college requires linguistic skills—namely, reading and writing—those with manual or artistic skills may be poor fits. The results of the emphasis on linguistic skills in our schools are twofold: Many students are not accepted by a college for enrollment or many accepted are flunked out of school before completion. The terms "flunk" or "fail," though referring to academic (i.e., linguistic) skills are perceived by students and parents alike to reflect upon the worth of the individual to whom these terms are directed.[17]

With a view toward preparation for college, parents concern themselves with their child's education. Placed high among the "subjects needed for college hierarchy" are mathematics, English, history, and science. One need not inquire as to the place of health instruction on some of these listings. Unfortunately, only upon dissatisfaction or disapproval will some parents' concerns be directed toward health education.

Note the sex education controversy. Parental involvement related to sex education can be described as either vituperative or consenting apathy. Parents seem to be vociferously opposed to sex education or conspicuously absent when meetings pertaining to sex education are held. Yet continual polling shows that about 80% of parents are in favor of sex education programs. Consequently, negative parental reactions regarding health education are prevalent forms of feedback received by school personnel associated with traditional health education programs.

In contrast, schools which allow their students to do volunteer work in hospitals or nursing homes, who involve students in their own learning to such a degree that these students are often speaking with excitement about health education, and who hire health educators as facilitators rather than as expositors of information find that the greatest allies of health instruction, second only to students, are the parents.

Getting students so excited about the health education they are experiencing that they express their exuberance to their parents and friends is the surest way of getting parental support for health education, and of aiding parents in realizing that a college education is not a prerequisite to establishing for oneself a significant and contributory role in our society.

CONCLUSION

An honest, though subjective, attempt has been made to describe the present status of health instruction. The reader who perceives a need for change of his or her instructional program need not feel forlorn. Only when the need for change is recognized can strategies be developed to result in properly directed adjustments. A recognized need, however, results in dissonance between what *is* being done and the readers' perceptions of what *ought* to be done. Consequently, such dissonance might very well result in a "bad-taste-in-the-mouth" attitude. Lest that persist, let me state that many fine health education programs are involving students and are examples to which health educators justifiably point with pride.[18,19,20] It is hoped that the reading of this book will create the *desire* for change, help the reader realize that change is *possible,* and present *methods* by which some of this needed change can be incorporated into health education programs.

Understandably, the reader will not be able to adopt a student-centered approach to health instruction in toto. Considering some inflexible school administrators, content-oriented students and parents, and a tradition of teacher-dominated instruction, to expect much change in a short period of time is unrealistic. However, there are many things which can be done *now*. For those desiring to move slowly toward an open type of health instructional process, the remainder of this book is recommended. The approach taken is one in which numerous instructional methodologies are offered—each of which is designed to activate the learner so as to expand the student's involvement in his or her own learning.

Hopefully, completely student-centered health education classes will someday be commonplace. In the meantime here's help in making your health instruction exciting, interesting, meaningful, and a showcase to be pointed to with pride.

REFERENCES

1. Fred Hein, Dana Farnsworth, and Charles Richardson, *Living: Health Behavior and Environment* (Glenview, Ill.: Scott, Foresman, 1970), p. 23.
2. Public Health Service, *Selected Vital and Health Statistics in Poverty and Non-poverty Areas of 19 Large Cities: United States, 1969–71* (U.S. Department of Health, Education, and Welfare, November 1975).
3. A notable exception is the objectives of health education as stated in the School Health Education Study, *Health Education: A Conceptual Approach: Experimental Curriculum Project* (Washington, D.C.: School Health Education Study, 1965).
4. Robert F. Mager, *Preparing Instructional Objectives* (Palo Alto, Calif.: Fearon, 1962), p. 47.
5. Ibid., p. 12.
6. John T. Fodor and Gus T. Dalis, *Health Instruction: Theory and Application* (Philadelphia: Lea & Febiger, 1966), p. 62.
7. For more detailed information about the Exchange the reader is referred to W. James Popham, "The Instructional Objectives Exchange: New Support for Criterion-Referenced Instruction," *Phi Delta Kappan,* Nov. 1970, pp. 174–175.
8. For example, New York State requires that health education be taught at the junior and senior high school level by a qualified health educator.
9. John Vaizey and Michael Debeauvais, "Economic Aspects of Educational Development;" *Education, Economy, and Society,* edited by A. H. Halsay, Jean Floud, and C. Arnold Anderson (New York: The Free Press, 1961), pp. 37–49.
10. Robert Fox and Kent Owen, "New Directions for Health Education Through Instructional Television," *The Journal of School Health,* April 1971, p. 188.

11. John T. Lawler, "Peer Group Approach to Drug Education," *Journal of Drug Education* **1** (1971), pp. 63–76.

12. Robert Goldhammer, *Clinical Supervision: Special Methods for the Supervision of Teachers* (New York: Holt, Rinehart, & Winston, 1969), p. 12.

13. Michigan Department of Education, *Patterns and Features of School Health Education in Michigan Public Schools* (Michigan: Department of Education, 1969), pp. 7–8.

14. American Alliance for Health, Physical Education, and Recreation, "AAHE Directory of Institutions Offering Specialization in Health Education," *School Health Review* **5** (1974), pp. 25–31.

15. J. Charles Jones, *Learning* (New York: Harcourt, Brace, & World, 1967), p. 72.

16. Walter Sorochan, "Health Instruction—Why Do We Need It in the '70s?," *The Journal of School Health,* April 1971, p. 209.

17. For more detailed discussions pertaining to this analysis the reader is referred to John Gardner's *Excellence* (New York: Harper & Row, 1961) and John Holt's *How Children Fail* (New York: Dell, 1964).

18. Wynette Hoffman, "The Short Life Line," *Journal of School Health* **46** (1976), p. 48.

19. David G. Bauer, "The Primary Prevention Project," *Health Education* **7** (1976), p. 9.

20. B. E. Pruitt, "The Open Contract—A Program of Individualized Study," *Health Education* **6** (1975), pp. 37–38.

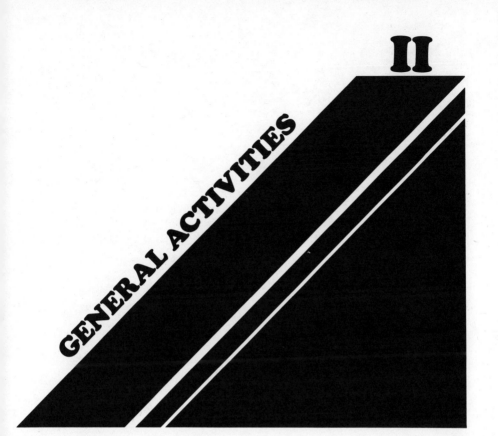

GENERAL ACTIVITIES

II

2

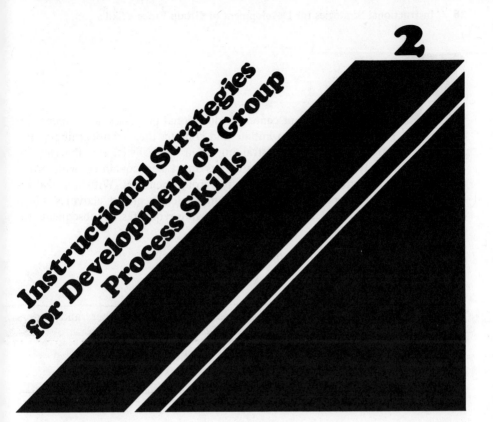

Instructional Strategies for Development of Group Process Skills

Requisite to student-centered educational processes are human relations skills. To expect students to initiate and conduct their own learning activities without prior human relations training seems unrealistic. For the class to function effectively as a group, the students must be acquainted with group dynamics and able to operate as productive group members. With this realization in mind, this chapter addresses itself to student-centered activities which can be used in classrooms to develop the following requisites to subsequent student-centered instruction:

1. Familiarity with and trust of other students in the class.
2. Friendship with at least one classmate.
3. Listening skills.
4. Knowledge of and experience with roles assumed by members and leaders of groups.
5. Knowledge of and experience with the decision-making process.
6. Cooperation and participation among all members of the class.
7. An understanding and appreciation of both one's own feelings and the feelings of others.
8. Open communication among disagreeing factions and empathy with those of opposing viewpoints.
9. Recognition of unfulfilled needs of students in the class and means of satisfying those needs.
10. Appreciation of individual differences and unique potentials.

EXERCISES FOR DEVELOPING REQUISITE SKILLS

Introduction Skits

If classes are to be conducted in an open, informal manner, and students are expected to verbally interact, the more each student knows about every other student, the better each student can evaluate what is being stated. It is often helpful to know where one stands when one speaks. Another point worth mentioning is that we tend to fear that which is strange to us. We are more likely to fear—or at least be uneasy with—things or people we don't know than those we do know. Prejudice is often a result of inaccurate generalizations directed at a strange people—people we don't know very well.

   To build trust among classmates, then, it is recommended that they know one another. Of course, one class period is not sufficient time for classmates to feel comfortable with one another. As the history of a class develops, however, trust can be developed—thereby enhancing an open, informal, verbally active class format. A beginning of this process can take several directions. It is possible for each student to stand up in class and mention a few facts or thoughts about him- or herself. It is possible for a classmate who knows a student to introduce that student to the class. However, a more interesting activity can be organized.

Divide the class into groups of six members each. With 20 minutes preparation time, each group is responsible for presenting a three-minute skit which will serve to introduce the members of that group. During the author's experience with this technique, several interesting skits were developed. One group role-played a drug raid, with one pupil a policeman who asked the others questions about their lives as he was searching them for drugs. Another group established one student as psychiatrist and the others as patients who one-by-one visited the psychiatrist's office to talk about their lives.

The teacher or the students may decide to associate a particular theme with the skits. For instance, when the author established a television show format as the theme for introduction skits, one group set three chairs on a table, another chair on the floor separated from the table, and three other chairs by a partition. When three female students sat on the three chairs, the "Dating Game" television format was used to introduce the actors to the class. Another group used a late-night talk show format with a host who had guests stopping by to be interviewed. Still another group adopted an interview of famous sports figures by a television sportscaster to help learn something about their group's members.

A variation of the approach outlined above would allow time for the class to direct questions at group members so as to get to know them better.

Pyramiding

Introduction skits serve to introduce class members to one another. Though these introductions are initially useful, their superficiality is evident, and further activity directed at getting to know one another is needed. There are several approaches to this end, but the one the author has found of most worth is pyramiding. In employing pyramiding, the students are asked to look at someone in the class that they know, then forget that person and choose someone they do not know very well to be their partner. Each pair is told that they are to discuss no other topic than themselves—their aspirations, family history, interests, etc. After 20 minutes of this, each pair is to combine with another pair to form quartets. On combining, each student must introduce his or her original partner to the new pair. Once these introductions have been made, the members of each quartet begin a free-wheeling discussion about themselves. After another 15 minutes, quartets can be combined to form octets (groups of eight), then these can become groups of 16, then 32, etc. . . . .

A variation of this approach is to be concerned with content as well as process by suggesting a topic to be discussed after introductions are made. The topic might be any health-related one in which the students might be interested. An example of this type of pyramiding might be helpful: The instructor requires students to form pairs and talk only about themselves for 10 minutes. At the conclusion of that time, the teacher asks the pairs to direct their discussion to the question: How can I be safer as a pedestrian (or any other health-education related topic)? After 15 minutes of discussing this issue, the original pair combines with another pair to form a quartet. The quartet members begin their discussion by talking only about themselves (*not* the health related topic) until they feel properly introduced. When they do feel comfortable with one another, they commence to discuss the content question. Pyramiding might also be used more than once so as to allow those students who hadn't met one another until groups of 8 or 16 were formed to meet one another in pairs or quartets.

The advantages of pyramiding over introduction skits are several. First, the one-to-one basis of the original pairing provides the opportunity for students to get to know someone and talk with that person confidentially. No one is eavesdropping and since the topic is limited to oneself, talking about oneself is perceived to be neither boastful nor in poor taste. Second, since each student is responsible for introducing his or her partner to another pair, he or she is required to pay attention to what that partner says, and will more readily ask for statements to be clarified. Third, group sizes of two and four provide for and necessitate verbal interaction among all the group members. And last, students exit pyramiding feeling secure in that class because they have gotten to know a number of their classmates in an informal, nonpressured setting. Class discussions and student-centered activities should then be more easily conducted and more educationally rewarding.

"Tell Me" Questions

While pyramiding is very helpful in establishing an atmosphere of trust in the classroom, it is only as good as the quality of the discussions in which students are engaged. The teacher may, therefore, decide to help students break from their shells of trivia and superficiality by providing them with questions to which the pairs, quartets, etc., must respond. As stated, these questions can be content oriented. However, questions related to the feelings of each student will better allow students to get to know one another. The reader can develop questions which would be appropriate to the pyramiding exercise. Questions like the following have been successfully used for this purpose:

1. Tell me something you like.
2. Tell me something you don't like.
3. Tell me something that makes you laugh.
4. Tell me something that makes you cry.
5. Tell me something that frightens you.

6. Tell me something that comforts you.
7. Tell me something you want to say to me.
8. Tell me something you don't want to say to me.

It seems evident that responses to questions like these will develop discussions of interest and accomplish the objective of establishing rapport among students in the class. It should be noted that each of these questions relates to the feeling level of the students. No right or wrong answers are possible. The usual "name, rank, and serial number" types of information are omitted, and the students are free to show what they wish of their inner selves, as well as their already evidenced exteriors. It should be emphasized throughout that anyone who feels threatened or severely uncomfortable participating in any of these activities is free to choose *not* to participate.

Paraphrasing

Though apparently concerned with one another, people have difficulty in listening. To be sure, they hear. But do they listen? This exercise will clearly demonstrate the lack of listening skills typical of students and, for that matter, most other people.

First though, what prevents listening? Most people are so concerned with what they want to say—and with how to word their thoughts—that they can't be bothered with listening to what is being said to them.

Other things prevent listening, too. When one is biased, one listens to and remembers those items which can be used to support that bias. Comments not in support of that bias are not remembered.

Emotions can also prevent one from listening adequately. Anger, fear, alarm, and numerous other emotions which might be provoked by a speaker can prevent the listener from listening accurately.

Speakers who don't define their terms, or who use terms inaccurately, can easily be misunderstood. The speaker who uses terms inappropriately can be understood if the listener asks for clarification of terms. However, in many instances either the listener applies his or her own definitions to the term or isn't provided the opportunity to ask for such clarification.

In any case, paraphrasing can be useful in highlighting listening difficulties and developing listening skills. The class is divided into groups of three students each, and the teacher presents a question to be answered in small group discussion. The question might be, "Should marijuana be legalized?" or "Is abortion moral?" or it might pertain to any other health content area. The small groups are to discuss this question for 20 minutes in the following manner: After the student's comments, subsequent speakers must first paraphrase what was said by the previous speaker—to that speaker's satisfaction—before they can make their comment. If the first speaker does not feel that the paraphrase is accurate, he or she repeats his or her original comments and the paraphraser must then attempt a new paraphrase. At the outset, students will have a great deal of difficulty in paraphrasing accurately due to any one or a combination of the reasons previously cited related to poor listening skills. To aid the students participating in this exercise, they should be told to begin whatever they say with the words, "In other words, you said. . . ."

After the question posed by the teacher is discussed for 20 minutes, there should be a five-minute discussion in the small groups pertaining to the purposes of the paraphrasing exercise. However, during this five-minute discussion, each speaker must continue to paraphrase each previous speaker in offering his or her comments.

At the conclusion of this exercise, a group discussion including the whole class should result in students understanding their difficulty in listening and desiring to develop more effective listening skills. A repetition of this exercise periodically throughout the class' history may also be required in order to provide sufficient practice in listening.

Another means of practicing listening requires the teacher to tape-record several television or radio commercials. After they have listened to these tape recordings, students can be asked questions to which they can respond correctly only if they have listened carefully to the recordings.

It should be noted that since listening has become such a lost art (if you doubt this statement conduct these exercises), several repetitions of these activities and periodic referral to them will be required to develop listening skill. However, unless the time is spent to develop this skill, the teacher cannot be assured that the students are really communicating with one another.

Written Conversations

The evident frustration which results when students engage in the paraphrasing exercise can be somewhat alleviated by use of paper-pencil conversations. When the class becomes engaged in an emotional discussion in which it appears that those advocating one position are not listening to those who advocate an opposing position, the teacher can reintroduce the paraphrasing exercise or have the class conduct their conversation in writing. This requires the teacher to pair off students (in the example above, students advocating opposing positions) who will not be allowed to talk at all. Each pair is to discuss the issue at hand, but only in writing. That is, when one wants to say something, he or she writes it and passes it to the other to read. In this manner, students can refer back to previous statements which, being written, are matters of record. Time is required to read and write each statement, so each must stop to think about both what the other has said and what he or she wants to say. Due to the time required in reading and writing statements, emotional reactions are limited, and more rational thoughts and logical ideas are presented and discussed.

A discussion of this technique by the total class can result in an underlining of those factors inhibiting listening to which previous reference has been made.

As with the paraphrasing exercise, written conversations can be repeated during the semester when a sharpening of listening skills seems necessary.

Fishbowl Roles of Group Members

Each group, in order to be successful in meeting its goals, must consist of group members willing to assume certain roles within the group's functioning. Group members who do not assume these roles adequately or who assume disruptive, nonproductive roles usually falter and create frustration for themselves and the rest of the members. It follows then that education about these roles and how best to performs them would be useful to any potential group member. One method by which to develop a knowledge of group roles is entitled the fishbowl technique.

The fishbowling of roles of group members is begun by selecting seven students who are willing to participate in a group discussion. These students are escorted out of the room but not allowed to talk with each other until given permission to do so by the teacher. While these seven students are out of the classroom, the teacher discusses the roles played by group members. The discussion relates to the information that appears on a handout to the class—a handout that contains the following:

In all groups, roles are played by the group's membership. We will be observing a group discussion and should be looking for evidence of the following roles being played:

Task roles

1. People who ask for or give information.
2. People who ask for or give opinions.
3. People who ask for clarification or elaboration.
4. People who initiate or continue work at hand.
5. People who keep a record of the group's discussions.
6. People who define the group's position or summarize so as to orient the group.

Task roles are directed specifically at solving the group's task, problem, or question.

Maintenance roles

1. People who make jokes.
2. People who follow others.
3. People who compromise.
4. People who help to settle arguments by two or more of the membership.
5. People who make sure all the members feel, and are, involved in the group's deliberations.

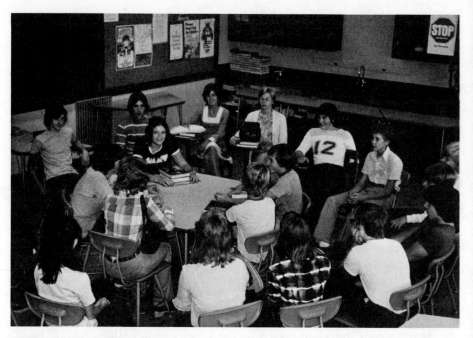

The fishbowl method requires an inner group surrounded by an outer group. A chair may be left empty as a means for outer-group students to enter the inner group's discussion.

Maintenance roles serve to keep the group cohesive, relieve frustration when necessary, and keep the members friendly toward one another. Though maintenance roles are not directly related to accomplishment of the group's task, without them task roles would not be effective.

Individual roles

1. People who want their own way all the time.
2. People who fool around too much.
3. People who attack others in the group.
4. People who always disagree.
5. People who say they are speaking for a larger group who are advocating a particular position.
6. People who continually interrupt others.

Individual roles block the group from effectively satisfying its goals and must therefore be minimized. As a group's history develops, successful groups have members increasingly playing task and maintenance roles with fewer and fewer individual roles being acted out.

As you observe a particular role being played in the group you will be observing, write down *exactly* what was said by the person playing that role.

The class is then seated around the periphery of the room with a smaller circle of chairs inside the larger one. The seven students who were not given the handout are then asked to reenter the classroom, sit in the chairs in the center of the room, ignore the rest of the class, and begin a discussion about anything they want. This discussion should last from 20 to 25 minutes and should not be interrupted by either the teacher or the other students. At the conclusion of this discussion, evidence should be presented by the student observers pertaining to the performance of particular group roles. Productive and nonproductive performances should be noted.

The following class session might be devoted to the practice of productive group roles in small group discussions with one or several student recorders assigned to each group to provide feedback on roles being played. Another way to practice positive group membership is to have an additional circle between the outside one (student observers) and inside one (group members). This additional circle would consist of students assigned to particular group members and to serve as coaches for those members; i.e., to help them be more productive and less disruptive. Further feedback can be provided, as before, by the outside circle of student observers. In any case, practice of effective group membership is necessary if, in subsequent classes concerned with content considerations, small groups will be formed to discuss issues and prepare reports of some kind.

Leadership Exercise

In each group at particular times, a leader either emerges or is appointed. Whether emergent or appointed (either by an authority figure like the teacher or by the group itself), a leader can better serve the group he or she leads by being aware of types of leadership and their associated levels of satisfaction and sense of achievement. To acquaint the students with these types of leadership, divide the class into small groups of six members each. Assign a leader for each group and meet at the front of the class briefly with all the leaders to explain to them the type of leadership they should exhibit. These leaders should be told to act authoritatively; i.e., to require members of the group to raise their hands and be acknowledged by the leader before speaking, to comment on the value (or lack of it) of each member's statement, and to eventually come to a decision for the group. Each leader is then given the following sheet to distribute to each of the members in his or her group:

DISCUSSION I

Rank the following eight traits in order of their importance for being a competent teacher. Place a number 1 by the most important, a number 2 by the second most important, and so on down to number 8, which will be the least important trait.

RANK	TRAIT
_____	tact
_____	honesty
_____	ambition
_____	courage
_____	warmth
_____	energy
_____	intelligence
_____	friendliness

After a 15-minute discussion, a group decision is required, and it will be communicated to the teacher by the leader. A record of the group's decision will also be kept by each of the group's members.

At the conclusion of Discussion I, a different student in each group is chosen leader and the new leaders meet with the teacher. The teacher defines their type of leadership as laissez-faire; i.e., they are to respond "I don't know" to questions, are not to call on anyone, and are not to be involved in the group's deliberations. The new leaders are then given the following sheet to distribute to each member of their group:

DISCUSSION II

Rank the following eight items in order of their importance for being a competent teacher. Place a number 1 by the most important, a number 2 by the second most important, and so on down to number 8, which will be the least important item.

RANK	ITEM
_____	A good understanding of the community.
_____	Ability to hold temper under aggravating circumstances.
_____	Ability to keep order in the classroom.
_____	Keeping parents informed of student's progress and development.
_____	Willingness to accept children whose standards and background differ radically from his or her own.
_____	Ability to make decisions based on fact rather than personal feelings.
_____	Ability to use time flexibly but still keep things moving.
_____	Ability to work with others.

After this 15-minute discussion, the decision arrived at and agreed to by the group will be communicated to the teacher and, as before, recorded and saved by each student.

At this point a third leader from each group is selected and told to act democratically; i.e., to attempt to hear from all group members, to offer his or her own opinion but not require that opinion to be accepted by the group, to be concerned with supplying task and maintenance roles when necessary, and to ensure consensual decision-making by the group. Each of these leaders are supplied the following sheets to distribute among their membership:

DISCUSSION III

Rank the following eight items in order of their importance for being a competent teacher. Place a number 1 by the most important, a number 2 by the second most important, and so on down to number 8, which will be the least important item.

RANK	*ITEM*
_____	**Talks effectively.**
_____	**Treats each student as an individual with unique abilities, interests, etc.**
_____	**Improves self by continuing formal education, reading current journals, attending workshops, training programs, etc.**
_____	**Relates well to other staff members.**
_____	**Brings in new ideas.**
_____	**Takes an active part in community affairs.**
_____	**Has ability to effectively handle administrative details.**
_____	**Is willing to try new techniques and methods.**

As before, each group's decision is related to the teacher and recorded by the group's members.

Upon completion of these three discussions (more than one day may be required), each student is asked to respond to the following items for *each* of the discussions:

1. How much satisfaction did you derive from the discussion?

   9 Completely satisfied
   8
   7 Moderately satisfied
   6
   5 Neutral; neither satisfied nor dissatisfied
   4
   3 Moderately dissatisfied
   2
   1 Completely dissatisfied

2. How much responsibility do you feel for the ranking you made as a group?

   9 Completely responsible
   8

7 Somewhat responsible
6
5 Neutral
4
3 Very little responsibility
2
1 Not responsible

3. How much hostility did you feel toward the leader?
9 No hostility
8
7 Some hostility
6
5 Neutral
4
3 A lot of hostility
2
1 Complete hostility

4. Rate the quality of the ranking you made as a group.
9 Best possible ranking.
8
7 Moderately good ranking
6
5 Average ranking
4
3 Moderately poor ranking
2
1 Worst possible ranking

The totals of the four responses are recorded and compared. The higher the score, the better the discussion. In most instances the democratic form of leadership will be preferred and the laissez-faire style of leadership liked least. A discussion of the reasons for these preferences will serve to reinforce democratic leadership when a leader is subsequently assigned or merges within a group in that class.

Lost on the Moon

Devised by Jay Hall, the "Lost on the Moon Game" is designed to help students learn to compromise and to take part in the consensual decision-making process. Consensual decision-making entails the agreement by group members about the decision reached. No voting or harrassing is allowed, and full discussion of all points of view is encouraged. Obviously this requires compromise and an inherent respect for other group members' opinions. Each student participating in the exercise is supplied with a copy of the following problem:*

> You are in a space crew originally scheduled to rendezvous with a mother ship on the lighted surface of the moon. Mechanical difficulties, however, have forced your ship to crashland at a spot some 200 miles from the rendezvous point. The rough landing damaged much of the equipment aboard. Since survival depends on reaching the mother ship, the most critical items available must be chosen for the 200-mile trip. The fifteen items left intact after the landing are listed below. Your task is to rank them in terms of their importance to your crew in its attempt to reach the rendezvous point. Place number 1 by the most important item, number 2 by the second most important, and so on through the least important, number 15.
>
> _____ Box of matches
>
> _____ Food concentrate
>
> _____ 50 feet of nylon rope
>
> _____ Parachute silk
>
> _____ Portable heating unit
>
> _____ Two .45 caliber pistols
>
> _____ One case dehydrated milk
>
> _____ Two 100-pound tanks of oxygen
>
> _____ Stellar map of the moon's constellation
>
> _____ Life raft containing CO_2 bottles
>
> _____ Magnetic compass
>
> _____ 5 gallons of water
>
> _____ Signal flares
>
> _____ First-aid kit containing injection needles
>
> _____ Solar-powered FM receiver-transmitter

The following is the correct ranking as determined by National Aeronautics and Space Administration (these are not distributed to the students at this point in the exercise):†

> 15 Box of matches (little or no use on the moon)
> 4 Food concentrate (supply daily food required)
> 6 50 feet of nylon rope (useful in taping injured, help in climbing)
> 8 Parachute silk (shelter against sun's rays)
> 13 Portable heating unit (useful only if party landed on dark side)
> 11 Two .45 caliber pistols (self-propulsion devices could be made from them)

---

* Special permission for reproduction of this material is granted by the author, Jay Hall, Ph.D., and publisher of Teleometrics International. All rights reserved and no reproductions should be made without express approval of Teleometrics International.

† Ibid.

12 One case dehydrated milk (food, mixed with water for drinking)
1 Two 100-pound tanks of oxygen (fills respiration requirement)
3 Stellar map of the moon's constellation (one of the principal means of finding direction)
9 Life raft (CO_2 bottles for self-propulsion across chasms, etc.)
14 Magnetic compass (probably no magnetized poles; thus, useless)
2 5 gallons of water (replenishes that lost in sweating, etc.)
10 Signal flares (distress call within line of sight)
7 First-aid kit containing injection needles (oral pills or injection medicine valuable)
5 Solar-powered FM receiver-transmitter (distress signal transmitter, possible communication with mother ship)

Each student is asked to rank the fifteen items individually in terms of importance. Groups of from six to eight students are then formed to rank the fifteen items as a group, utilizing consensual decision-making rather than voting or allowing one group member's opinion to override the group's. An analysis of individual and group opinions should reveal the advantage of consensual decision-making over decisions made by individuals.

To make such an analysis, the students first compute the difference between the NASA rankings and their individual rankings. For example, let's say that one of the boys in the class chooses the box of matches as number 1. The NASA ranking is 15, so the difference between the NASA ranking and the individual ranking is 14. The boy goes on to rank each item, then compares his rankings with those made by NASA. For each item he writes down the difference between the two rankings; then he adds up those differences to get his individual score in the same way. The lower the scores, of course, the greater the agreement between the individual's ranking and the NASA ranking.

Next, the ranking of the group as a whole is compared with the NASA ranking. That is, if the group utilizing consensual decision-making ranked the matches as number 12, whereas the NASA ranking is 15, the difference between that and the NASA ranking is only 3. As with the individual scores, the group score is calculated by totaling the differences.

Finally, the students compare their individual scores with the group score. In almost all cases, the group score will be lower—and therefore more accurate—than the individual score. This, of course, indicates that group decisions made consensually are likely to be better than those made individually. And this fact highlights the usefulness of participation and cooperation in groups.

Cooperation Exercise

Group members sometimes need to have the importance of cooperation emphasized. For the teacher to speak to the group of the need for the members to cooperate may sometimes be helpful. However, a more dramatic and effective method is available to make this point. The teacher prepares envelopes containing parts of a large square (like a jigsaw puzzle). An oak tag (manila) sheet of paper cut into variously shaped pieces can be used for this exercise. The class is asked what cooperation means. Some of the following points may be made:

a. Everyone has to understand the problem.
b. Everyone needs to believe that he or she can help.
c. Instructions have to be clear.
d. Everyone needs to think of the other person as well as himself or herself.

The class is then divided into small groups of four students each and given the following instructions:

> Each member of your group has an envelope containing parts of a square. When all the pieces in one group are placed properly together, like a jigsaw puzzle, they will form one large square with no pieces left over. Your task as a group is to form this large square. However, in accomplishing this task, no communication will be allowed, either verbal or nonverbal. You will not be allowed to *take* a piece of the puzzle from another group member; but you can *offer* another group member any one of your puzzle pieces that you wish.

Upon completion of this exercise, the teacher can ask the following questions:

1. How did you feel when someone held a piece and did not see the solution?
2. How did you feel about having to depend on others?
3. Were some people more cooperative than others?

Another means of demonstrating the need for cooperation in the class has employed five squares shaped as shown in Fig. 2.1. The squares are cut along the lines within them and the lettered pieces placed in separate envelopes as follows:

envelope 1: a,a,a,c
envelope 2: a,j,d
envelope 3: g,i,f,c
envelope 4: b,e,f,h

The students are then divided into groups of four, each group member receiving an envelope and a handout sheet on which appear the following directions:

> As of this moment you are not allowed to talk with one another nor communicate in any nonverbal fashion (no gesturing, making facial expressions, etc.). Pass out the envelopes so that each person has one in front of him or her. Take the pieces out and place the envelopes to one side. At a signal, the task of each group is to form five squares of equal size. This is

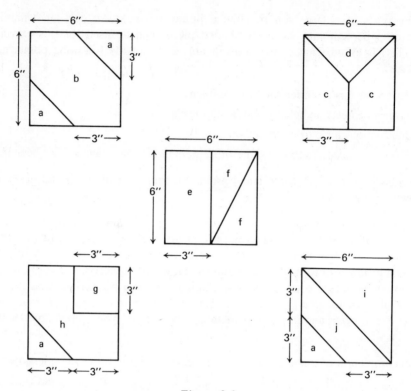

Figure 2.1

not a race, but the task is not completed until each group has before it five perfect squares of equal size.

You are not allowed to take or ask for a piece of the puzzle which is in front of someone else. You *are* allowed to give someone else a piece of the puzzle which is in front of you.

This exercise results in students realizing that cooperation often means giving of oneself and not only taking from the group. As with many of this type of exercise, the students will have fun while learning this very valuable lesson.

Still another means for demonstrating the importance of cooperation and, in particular, the negative aspects of competition within the group, is the "Win As Much As You Can"[1] game. Each participant is asked to pair off with another participant, and then, with that partner and three other pairs, to form a group of four pairs. With partners seated next to each other, and with the pairs squared off (as in square dancing), the seating formation appears as follows, with each participant facing the center of the square:

```
      A  A
  D        B
  D        B
      C  C
```

The narrator gives each participant a copy of the handout shown in Fig. 2.2, then reads the following instructions to the group:

The name of this game is 'Win As Much As You Can.' The objective is the same as the title—you are to try to win as much as you can. There will be

4X = lose $1.00	
3X	win $1.00
1Y =	lose $3.00
2X	win $2.00
2Y =	lose $2.00
1X	win $3.00
3Y =	lose $1.00
4Y = win $1.00	

Round	Time for Consultation	Vote	Won or Lost	Balance	Multiplication Factor
1	1 min. (partner)				
2	1 min. (partner)				
3	1 min. (partner)				
4	3 min. (group) 1 min. (partner)				3
5	1 min. (partner)				
6	1 min. (partner)				
7	3 min. (group) 1 min. (partner)				5
8	1 min. (partner)				
9	1 min. (partner)				
10	3 min. (group) 1 min. (partner)				10
			Total		

Figure 2.2

ten rounds of balloting. In every round, before voting, the two members of each pair will discuss with each other *only* how that pair's *one* vote for that round will be cast, X or Y. Consult the handout you were given for help in making a decision, X or Y. After each round's voting, find out how the other pairs voted and then consult the handout you have for distribution of money. As you go along, keep a tally of how much your pair has won or lost during each round and the total amount won or lost up to that point in the game. As you can see on your handout, some rounds' winnings are multiplied so that if the scoring box indicates you won $3.00, for instance, you would multiply that amount by that round's multiplication factor. There will be rounds when you will be allowed to consult with the three other pairs in your group before you vote, and to make any arrangements with them that you would like. I will remind you when those rounds appear. Now you have one minute to consult with your partner before casting your pair's ballot for round number one.

At the end of the ten rounds the teacher places the totals of each pair on the chalkboard so that each group's pairs are separate from the other groups' pairs. For example:

Group 1	Group 2	Group 3
−18	+52	+35
−37	−41	−26
+5	−25	−5
−2	−10	−13

The instructor then initiates a discussion among the class members which revolves around the following questions:

1. What did "Win as much as you can" mean to you?
2. Who should have won as much as they could? Each pair? Each group? The total of all the groups?
3. How did you feel when the competition became intense?

After the discussion, the instructor should then add up the total amount of money won or lost by each group (for instance, Group 1 lost $52.00, Group 2 lost $24.00, and Group 3 lost $9.00) and tell the class that if each pair had chosen to vote Y each round, each pair would have won $25.00 and the group would have won $100.00. A vote of Y would have been best for all and could be considered a "cooperative vote." Transfer should be made from this game to the necessity of cooperation in the classroom and in small groups within the classroom.

Baseball Clue Game

Often in classes, several students dominate during verbal discussion. It could be that those students are "pushy," or it could be that the silent class members feel they have nothing worthwhile to contribute. In either case, the Baseball Clue Game should help broaden the pattern of communication in the class.

Each player gets an index card on which a clue is written. Since there are only seventeen clue cards, the class will have to be divided in half and two sets of clue cards will be needed (one for each group). No player may let anyone else read his or her clue but may verbally relate that clue to the others in that group. The clues, of course, are needed to solve the problem, and therefore each student rightfully feels that he or she has something of worth to contribute. Teachers can make up their own problems and clues, but a sample relating to baseball follows:

Problem:

What are the names of the players on the baseball team and which positions do they play?

Clues:

The shortstop, the third baseman, and Bill each won $100 betting on the fight.

Harry and the third baseman live in the same building.

Jerry is taller than Bill.

Paul and Allen each won $20 from the pitcher at pinochle.

One of the outfielders is either Mike or Andy.

Mike is shorter than Bill. Each of them is heavier than the third baseman.

Sam is involved in a divorce suit.

Paul, Andy, and the shortstop each lost $50 at the race track.

Ed and the outfielders play poker during their free time.

All the battery and infield, except Allen, Harry, and Andy, are shorter than Sam.

The pitcher's wife is the third baseman's sister.

Ed's sister is engaged to the second baseman.

Paul, Harry, Bill, and the catcher took a trouncing from the second baseman at pool.

Andy dislikes the catcher.

Ed, Paul, Jerry, the right fielder, and the center fielder are bachelors. The others are married.

The catcher and the third baseman each have two children.

The center fielder is taller than the right fielder.

Solution:

Harry is the pitcher.

Allen is the catcher.

Paul is the first baseman.

Jerry is the second baseman.

Andy is the third baseman.

Ed is the shortstop.

Sam is the left fielder.

Mike is the right fielder.

Bill is the center fielder.

Once the class is accustomed to the clue game technique, the teacher might want to vary the technique for specific purposes. For example, there may be a group of verbally active students and another group of verbally inactive students in the class. The teacher could then give clues only to the quiet students and have them seated in a circle in the center of the room working out the solution, while each of the other students is seated behind a quiet student and acting as a coach for that student. In this exercise, only the "inner circle" students are allowed to speak to the large group, while the "outer circle" students (usually very verbal) are limited to only communication with the person behind whom they are sitting.

A periodic repeat of these communication techniques is recommended. Some students need to participate in several exercises of this kind before they can feel comfortable enough in a class to speak up without hesitation when they feel they have something worthwhile to contribute.

Role Reversal

Role playing is often used to develop a sense of empathy for particular people. For example, a student who has evidenced a bias against negroes may be asked by the teacher to act the part of a black in a role-playing situation. It is hoped that putting a student in another's shoes will help that student to develop an understanding of the other person's situation. Similarly, role playing might be employed to help students to empathize with parents of teenage children. In using role playing in this manner, a student might be asked to act the part of a parent whose teenage daughter, played by another student, returns from a date two hours past her curfew. Playing the role of parents will help students develop a greater appreciation for the parent's "side of the coin," and increased empathy for parents. It demonstrates the complexity of seemingly uncomplicated situations which occur between parents and children.

Likewise, role reversal can develop empathy between those advocating opposing points of view. In the example cited above, parents could be invited to school and asked to play the role of child, while their child plays the role of parent. In this manner parent and child should better appreciate one another's point of view.

In the context of this chapter, however, role reversal is suggested as a means of developing more effective groups. It is desirable for two members of a group who are disagreeing with each other to reverse roles so as to develop an appreciation of the opponent's point of view. Compromise will be more easily achieved and more palatable if each group member is able to perceive some validity in each opposing viewpoint. At still other points in the group's existence, particular members might be dysfunctional in the group due to any one of a number of reasons: boredom, need for attention, aggressive nature, or a dislike of the group's members, for example. In these instances it is wise to provide feedback to the disruptive group member relative to his or her behavior. One effective manner in which to provide this feedback is through the role reversal technique. The dysfunctional student can be asked to act the role of the leader of the group while another student portrays the dysfunctional student. An awareness of their behavior and its effect upon the leader of the group is often all that is needed for group members to behave in a productive manner. For fear of forgetting the nature of role reversal, it should be noted that an appreciation for the needs of individuals within the group is the responsibility of the group leader and is enhanced in the role reversal example just cited.

There are other ways to respond to dysfunctional group members. Either an audio or videotape recording might be employed and analyzed to document disruptive behavior. However, one of the most effective manners of relating to a student who has been demonstrating antigroup behavior is to have each group member act like any other group member of his or her choosing while the others try to guess who he or she is acting like. Often this technique causes the dysfunctional group member to realize how disruptive he or she has been. A discussion by the group about the feelings each student had when he or she was being portrayed by someone else will help to limit dysfunctional group behavior.

One other very effective manner for helping the group deal with such behavior requires first that the group stand in a circle. Each student then takes a turn to stand in front of each other student, hold his or her hand, look the person in the eyes, and reveal feelings about that person. Only the student going around the circle may speak until the exercise is over. At this point, explanations about the reasons for these feelings will often reveal to dysfunctional students what effect their behavior has on others in the group and how they feel about them. It is suggested that no more than eight students form a circle and that, before asking the students to divulge their feelings, the teacher highlight the differences between feelings (see the mental health chapter) and thoughts.

Other means of responding to disruptive or dysfunctional behavior include assigning such a student a particular role to play in the group. Such roles might be recorder, summarizer, or clarifier (see "Fishbowl Roles of Group Members" in this chapter), so that the student experiences and practices constructive group behavior.

Filling Needs

This appropriately named exercise is another which can be employed to help leaders of groups to fill the needs of problem members in an effective manner. A seemingly simple exercise, this activity is one of the most valuable in a group leader's repertoire. Each group member is asked to make a list in response to the question, "What can we do to make you happier in this group?" Upon completion of the lists, each group member can read his responses to the question while others react to his individual needs. Another possibility is for the leader to collect the responses and assign group members to help fill the needs of other group members. In any case, it is important to realize that groups are most effective when the needs of their members are satisfied.

Appreciation of Individual Differences

In spite of what students list as their needs as group members, an appreciation of their individuality may be all that is needed to make them productive group members. Students who join a group often neglect the individual and his or her uniqueness and exalt the group. The author has found it helpful in these instances to conduct an exercise which begins with a reading of the following excerpt:[2]

> In all my years of teaching, Charlie McCaffrey was the finest student I ever had. Charlie failed most of the tests I gave him; he very seldom finished his science homework; he struggled for C's and generally got D's; but Charlie McCaffrey was the finest student I ever taught. No matter how I tried to impress Charlie with the contributions of Kepler and Newton, he could just never take them seriously. But ask for a volunteer to adjust the blinds, feed the fish, or clean out the snake cage and Charlie was on his feet and moving.
>
> I always felt like a rat giving Charlie a C (and that was really a charitable act); the kid was just too much a nice guy. He was never mad at anyone. He always smiled. And his red hair always dropped into his left eye, which gave him an excuse to be inattentive just when I was trying to make a critical point about how he hadn't even tried to grasp the contribution of Gregor Mendel. That kid! What a pain! He just didn't take science seriously.
>
> Like the time I had a really important test. I told the class, well in advance, "This is important. It's critical to your mark." Charlie bombed it. I mean a flat F. But what can you say to a kid you like who failed your test? It was a time when "Charlie the Tuna" ads were in full swing on television. I didn't want to be too rough, so I drew a fishing line down through his paper and attached a note to the hook, which just said, "Sorry, Charlie." His mother had been a teacher and a lot of her friends were teachers. When he took the paper home they laughed and understood. I mean, she had to live with this kid who just didn't appreciate that Tycho Brahe had a gold nose.
>
> In retrospect, I realize that Charlie was the kind of person the world needs more of. His temperament was equable. The sparkle of enthusiasm enlivened

his eye. He never deviated from his way of life. He was the perfect public relations man, promoter, communicator, a potential contributor to society. And I gave him a C.

So, Charlie, you said I was your favorite teacher, the guy who treated everyone as if he was unique. But you were out of my class. I said I individualized, but in your case I didn't. What a great mayor of Boston you would have made!

I won't make the same mistake again. When, if ever, another Charlie comes along I'll be ready. I was sorry, Charlie, when you were killed in Viet Nam. I spent all that time trying to change you—and you changed me.

I'll say it again. I'm sorry, Charlie.

Following the reading, there is a discussion of the meaning of this excerpt and the lesson's transferability to each student's group. Next, the teacher reads the following two case studies and asks the students to classify the future of the two people described as hopeful, unpredictable, or hopeless.

Case 1 This boy is a senior in high school and has obtained a certificate from a physician stating that a nervous breakdown necessitates his leaving school for six months. The teacher describes this boy as a problem. He is not a good all-around student, has no friends, spoke late as an infant, and his father is ashamed of his son's lack of athletic ability. This boy has odd mannerisms, has made up his own religion, and chants hymns to himself.

Case 2 This six-year-old boy's head was large at birth and he was therefore thought to have brain fever. Three of his siblings died before birth but the mother disagrees with relatives and neighbors who insist the child is abnormal. When the child is sent to school, however, he is diagnosed as mentally ill. This diagnosis infuriates the mother who withdraws the boy from school and says she will teach him herself.

After these case studies have been presented and the two children's futures have been determined to be either hopeful, unpredictable, or hopeless, the teacher then announces that the person discussed in the first case was Thomas Edison and the one in the second case was Albert Einstein. Obviously, the point is then made that each person is unique with the potential for considerable contribution and that this uniqueness should be appreciated and rewarded in the group.

Trust Test

For groups to be effective, group members must trust one another. The development of trust is the point of this whole section. The particular exercise herein described, however, will afford the teacher the opportunity to test trust in the group. With the class preferably seated in a circle, each student thinks of a problem or secret which he or she does not usually share with others. Without relating that secret to the group, each student goes around the circle telling the class how he or she thinks each other student would respond if they did tell the secret. In this manner, the degree to which each student is trusted by the group is readily perceived.

Trust Walk

Another manner in which to test trust or to develop trust initially, is known as the Trust Walk. In this exercise, students are paired with other students they don't know very well. Each pupil is then asked to share a concern with his or her partner in conversation. After 10 minutes of conversing, each pair is asked to take a walk for 20 minutes. The first 10 minutes of the walk, one partner must keep his or her eyes closed and is not allowed to talk to the other student who is leading. After 10 minutes the leader and "blind walker" reverse roles. On return, each pair shares its feelings about the exercise. Those who have participated in trust walks often mention that their feeling of trust increased as the walk progressed.

Color Jigsawing

Often in groups, the creative potential of group members is thwarted and frustration develops. However, frustration can develop for numerous reasons and its manifestation can take many forms. This exercise, done with colored pieces of poster board of various shapes, illustrates reactions to the limitation of creativity and to frustration. On its completion, ways to respond to these reactions are discussed.

Students are seated around tables—six to twelve students to each table. On each table are different colored and different shaped pieces of poster board, cut out prior to class by the teacher, in sufficient number so that each student can create a design to his or her desire. After they have had 15 minutes of creating designs with the colored poster board pieces, the students are instructed to dismantle their designs and to adhere to the following instructions:

1. Take the long red piece in your right hand.
2. Take the round yellow piece in your left hand.
3. Place the red piece adjacent and to the left of the yellow piece.
4. Now pick up a small white piece.
5. etc.

The instructions continue for 20 minutes. After approximately 10 minutes, frustration reactions begin to surface. One student may yawn (withdrawal behavior), another student may protest the absurdity of the exercise (rationalization), a third student may disrupt the situation (attack reaction), and still an-

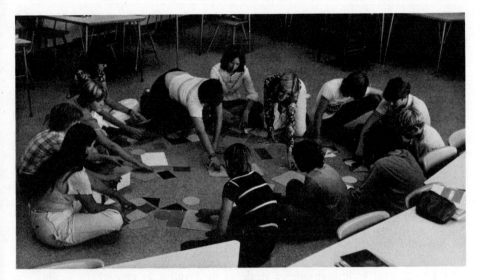

These students are doing Color Jigsawing with poster board.

other student may resort to laughter and playing (regressive behavior). After the instructions have elicited the above reactions, a discussion of how people respond to frustration will serve to help students recognize frustrated group members. Further discussion might determine how the group should react to frustrated group members (filling needs, for example).

Building-Upon Exercise

One of the more serious, but correctable, examples of group dysfunction is that of group members failing to respond to what has been said. Rather, students are anxious to add new and often unrelated remarks. A well-functioning group builds upon each member's contribution so that the end product of that group is the collective and interrelated thoughts and ideas of its members. Such collective material is most often better than a pooling of individual ideas.

One manner in which to help groups practice building upon each other's ideas is to structure a group discussion so that after Speaker 1 has reacted to a question posed by the teacher, Speaker 2 must cite all the ways in which he or she agrees and disagrees with what Speaker 1 has said. Speaker 3 then responds to Speaker 2 in similar fashion, and so on until everyone in the group has had a turn. A discussion of the difficulty in not being allowed to add new ideas, and in identifying points of agreement and disagreement, will prepare the group for the next phase of this exercise.

For that phase, have the students discuss a new problem but allow them to add new ideas *after* they cite points of agreement and disagreement as they did before. This discussion should be structured as the previous one; i.e., Speaker 2 responds to Speaker 1, Speaker 3 to Speaker 2, etc.

Group Disagreement Game

In any group's history there are times when there is a great deal of disagreement on a particular issue. Two techniques have been demonstrated to be of great value at these particular times. The first technique requires the group to discuss the issue about which they are disagreeing—but before offering comments the student speaking must first cite those aspects of the previous speaker's comments with which he or she agrees. All speakers therefore begin their comments on a positive note; e.g., "I agree with you that . . . ," rather than immediately disagreeing with what has been stated. In addition, while listening to others speaking, the listener must be attuned to viewpoint ideas with which he or she and the speaker are in agreement rather than only those about which they differ.

The second technique allows students to develop an empathetic feeling for those with whom they disagree and a better understanding of opposing points of view. This activity requires that those in disagreement switch positions so that they are, in effect, arguing for the position with which they disagree. By way of example, if student A is opposed to legalization of marijuana and is arguing with student B who favors its legalization (or decriminalization), the teacher requests that for a short period of time student A argue for legalization and student B against it (just the opposite of their actual opinions). Having to think of cogent arguments for a position you disagree with results in a better understanding of that position and greater appreciation for those favoring that position.

CONCLUSION

The activities and exercises described in this chapter are recommended for use throughout a health education class' experience, but particularly at the beginning of the term. In this way, such skills as listening, communicating, and cooperating; dealing with frustration, group dysfunction, and disagreement; and the development of trust, personal worth, and camaraderie can be accomplished early and serve as prerequisites to health content considerations. These coping skills are essential in life. As will be obvious, the development of the skills, feelings, and group atmosphere referred to in this chapter will be necessary for a successful experience with the learning activities described in subsequent chapters.

It should be noted that small-group work need not command all of the class time. Large-group instructional activities can be vehicles for meaningful learning experiences as well. Small groups do, however, provide greater opportunity for students to be active in the learning process and therefore should be employed on a regular basis.

One last word: The activities described have been employed with success by both the author and many school teachers who have been enrolled in his classes. The delight experienced after students complete these exercises is so rewarding that students and teacher alike will wonder what their schooling has meant to this point, and look forward to the next day's health class with anticipation.

REFERENCES

1. This exercise is based on the work of William Gellermann and adapted from J. William Pfeiffer and John E. Jones, *Structured Experiences for Human Relations Training, Volume II* (Iowa City, Iowa: University Associates Press, 1970), pp. 66–69. Used by permission.
2. Victor J. Gerhard, Jr. "Sorry Charlie . . . ," *Phi Delta Kappan* **53,** 8 (1972), p. 536. Used by permission.

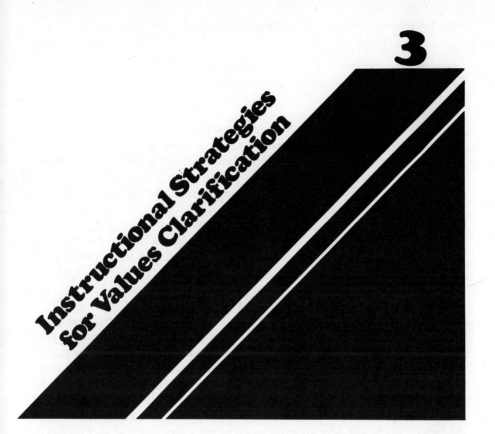

3

Instructional Strategies
for Values Clarification

This chapter offers the teacher exercises with which to help students clarify their values. A knowledge of where one is seems important before one proceeds to journey anywhere. Therefore, the classroom activities included in this chapter are directed at establishing, for students, the point from which they are beginning their educational journey. A reintroduction to these activities at the end of the academic semester or year will serve to determine the changes in values associated with that time period.

It should be noted that the activities included in this values clarification section are not directed at *developing* values. Rather, they seek to create awareness on the part of the student regarding values already possessed. Changes in values may then be deemed appropriate by the student, and the teacher's help in changing particular values may be sought.

Since our decisions are based on the values system we share, the exploration of our values seems a necessity. To make more rational decisions relative to our health and health-related behavior, we must understand ourselves and our motivations. A study of the values we possess will contribute to such an understanding. As with all the other exercises described in this book, the teacher should be lucid on the rationale for incorporating values clarification activities in the health instructional process. Much harm can be done to the movement for humanistic health education by teachers who play "games" in the classroom without an understanding of how those "games" contribute to the growth and development of the children participating in these activities. Although such teachers usually tend to revert to more traditional health instruction, observers (parents, school administrators, etc.) are apt to generalize the ineffectiveness of humanistic health education to other situations. Consequently, instructors who employ humanistic education effectively are likely to be viewed with some suspicion.

Values are determined through the use of three processes:

1. Choosing
   a. freely
   b. from alternatives
   c. after thought given to the consequences of each alternative

---

Much of this chapter and the valuing activities in subsequent chapters derive from Louis Raths, Merrill Harmin, and Sidney Simon, *Values and Teaching: Working with Values in the Classroom* (Columbus, Ohio: Charles E. Merrill, 1966) and the subsequent work of Sidney Simon. For information about current values clarification materials or a series of nationwide workshops, contact the National Humanistic Education Center, 110 Spring St., Saratoga Springs, N.Y. 12866.

2. Prizing
   a. satisfied with the choice
   b. willing to announce the choice publicly
3. Acting
   a. actually behaving consistent with the choice
   b. part of a general pattern of life[1]

Unless all nine of the criteria for valuing (the three categories and their subcategories) are met, the item in question is not a value. It may be a belief, opinion, or attitude, but not a value. An example here might serve to clarify this point. If one professes to value good health and has thought about the implications of and alternatives to good health (choosing criterion), is happy with that choice and talks with others about it (prizing criterion), but doesn't behave in a healthy manner by not exercising regularly (acting criterion), then good health is not a *value* for that person.[2]

VALUING EXERCISES

The exercises that follow are directed at identifying for the students the nature and direction of their values. Consequently, the three valuing processes are the subject of these activities.

Values Ranking

An activity which can help students to set priorities of values is to have them rank circumstances according to their preference *for* those circumstances. For example, rank the following situations with number 1 being the most preferred, 2 the second most preferred, and 3 the least preferred:

1. To drop a napalm bomb on a village in Southeast Asia knowing that scores of innocent people will be killed and injured.
2. To press the button which will activate an electric chair in which a convicted killer is sitting.
3. To press down on the accelerator of your car, thereby running down and killing three men coming at you on a dark night with crowbars.

Analysis of the ranking above proves useful relative to values pertaining to life. Though professing to value life above all else, those selecting choice 3 as most preferable may actually mean their *own* life. Those selecting choice 2, in which only one person is killed, may be those who actually do value life above all else. Students selecting choice 1 as most preferable may do so because of the distance from the results of their action. Obviously, other conclusions relative to values can be obtained utilizing this exercise.

Below are other groupings which may be used in value ranking:

1. disfigurement	1. charming	1. African Negro
2. loss of intelligence	2. reliable	2. Mexican Negro
3. poverty	3. insightful	3. American Negro
1. Jewish	1. preschooler	1. drug pusher
2. Christian	2. teenager	2. drug addict
3. Atheist	3. adult	3. drug grower

Values Grid

Similar to values ranking, in that students have to set priorities, the value grid allows for more than three rankings at one time. Students are asked to draw a grid consisting of four cells across and four cells down, to total 16 cells (Fig. 3.1). The first column will be labeled "Very Strong," the second "Strong," the third "Mild," and the last column, "No Opinion." The teacher reads 16 statements, one at a time, thus: first the statement, then identification for the students of the key word in the statement, then a few seconds pause. During this

Very Strong	Strong	Mild	No Opinion

Fig. 3.1   Values Grid

pause, students are to categorize the statement just read by how strongly they feel about the statement—regardless of whether they favor it or oppose it.

When the 16 statements have been read, each and every cell in the grid will contain one, and only one, *key word* which refers to a particular statement. It's important to remember that whether a student feels *very strongly in favor of* or *very strongly opposed to* a statement, the key word describing that statement should be placed in one of the four cells in the "Very Strong" column. When all statements have been categorized, the grid will contain four key words in each of its four columns. The class is then divided into groups of four, who are to discuss the grids of each of their group's members. Reasons for choices should be stressed and personal experiences relative to the statements recalled.

Although teachers can develop their own sets of statements, the following statements, with the key words in italics, have been used successfully:

1. A teacher calls a student *dumb* in front of the class.
2. A senior boy tries to *seduce* as many girls in the sophomore class as he can in order to prove his manliness.
3. Someone has seen a person they know rifling *lockers* but doesn't tell anyone.
4. A girl is asked to *lie* for another student.
5. A girl has become *promiscuous* trying to be popular.
6. A boy does not want to participate in the *draft*.
7. A student is suspended for *smoking*.
8. A student is thrown out of class for *cheating*.
9. An unwed mother is advised by a friend to have an *abortion*.
10. A student decides to leave home because he doesn't have enough *freedom*.
11. A pot missionary gives *pot* to others because he thinks it is a cure-all.
12. A student is playing the game of applying to *college* because of parental pressure.
13. A student behaves differently with different groups in order to get *elected* student body president.
14. A student *shoplifts* as part of a fraternity (sorority) initiation.
15. Parents *beat* their daughter if she disobeys them.
16. A student was thrown out of class because she wasn't wearing a *bra*.

Values Continuum

Many people will proclaim the value they ascribe to seat belts in automobiles. Surprisingly, many people, though valuing seat belts, will not wear them. The Values Continuum is useful in helping us see the inconsistencies between what we profess to be our values and how we behave. Relative to seat belts, the reader is asked to place himself or herself at the appropriate place on the following continuum:

How often do you wear seat belts?

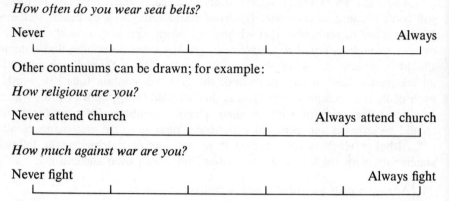

Other continuums can be drawn; for example:

How religious are you?

How much against war are you?

From these continuums, discussions relative to student behavior can be developed and suggestions for more consistent behavior with professed values elicited.

Activities Enjoyed

Another useful activity to clarify the acting-out aspect of values requests students to list 20 things they enjoy doing. It is surprising how difficult a task this is in itself. After the list is complete the following instructions may be presented:

1. Place a dollar sign next to each item which cannot be done without an initial outlay of at least five dollars.
2. Place a "P" next to those items which you prefer to do with other people and an "A" next to those things you prefer to do alone.
3. Place a "5" next to any item which you would not have listed 5 years ago.
4. Place a "G," for generation gap, next to each item which your parents would not have included on their list.
5. Think of a person you love, and place an "L" next to each item you would want that person to include on his or her list.
6. Place an "M" next to the five items on the list which you *most* enjoy.
7. Record the date when you last did each of the items you just marked with an "M."

An activity of this sort shows whether or not those things most enjoyed are those things most often done, how values may change, how materialistic one may be, and how different generations may or may not possess similar values. Of course, several other interpretations may develop during a discussion of this exercise with the students.

An important aspect of this exercise, as well as of other values clarification activities, is that it does not force the teacher's values on the students in the class. All that is required is that the students analyze for themselves what they think they value and how they behave relative to their perceived values. Students then will have to choose between acting more consistently with their own desired values, or changing their perceptions of those values to be more in line with desirable behaviors.

Coat of Arms

By learning more about themselves and sharing a little of themselves with others, students will be better prepared to make decisions pertaining to use of drugs, choice of marriage partner, choice of occupation, etc. The assumption is that the more one knows about oneself, the more one's motivations for behavior are recognizable and accounted for in the decision-making process. To help in this respect, students are asked to do the following:

1. On a large sheet of paper draw the shape you see in Fig. 3.2—but *do not* write in the numbers. Draw the figure as large as you can, because you will be adding pictures or words to each of the six sections.
2. In Section 1, draw two pictures: one showing something you are very good at, and the other showing something you're not very good at but would like to do better.
3. In Section 2, draw a picture depicting one value to which you are deeply committed.
4. In Section 3, draw a picture representing the material possession which is most dear to you.
5. In Section 4, draw two pictures: one describing your greatest accomplishment during the past year, and the other representing your biggest failure during the past year.

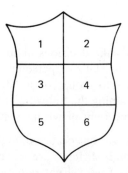

Figure 3.2

6. For Section 5, assume you had one year to do whatever you wanted and were guaranteed success. Draw a picture in Section 5 representing the activity you would choose to do for that year.

7. Finally, in Section 6, write three words which you would want others to use in describing you if you were to die today.

On completing these seven steps, each student will have a coat of arms. Students should be encouraged to share their coats of arms in small-group discussion at this point. In this manner, students will learn more about themselves and their classmates.

Values Quadrant

Still another exercise which can be employed for student self-analysis begins with a large square containing four quadrants. In the upper left quadrant students are to list 10 people with whom they would like to be friends or with whom they are friends. In the lower left section, students are asked to list 10 places that they like to go; i.e., 10 places where they enjoy spending their time.

In the upper right section the student should list five people with whom he or she does not want to be friends; people he or she doesn't like. Lastly, in the lower right space, the student should list five places at which he or she does not enjoy spending time.

The completed quadrants can then be examined and discussed or analyzed separately by each student. Questions should then be related to why certain people are liked and others disliked; why certain places are enjoyed and others are not; what would happen to the places enjoyed if the people that are disliked went to them; how would the people that are liked be viewed if they were associated with places that are not enjoyed; and how people and places can be transformed from the right-hand side of the quadrant (disliked people and unenjoyed places) to the left-hand, or positive side. How often people who are liked are taken to places that are liked is still another question which serves to help students analyze their Values Quadrants.

Who Should Survive?

When students are asked to make decisions about the relative worth of people, the value ascribed to particular skills or personality attributes surfaces. For this exercise, the class is divided into groups of six students each, and each student is given a handout sheet containing the following information (the teacher should make it clear that there are no right or wrong answers as such):

Survival Problem An atomic war has occurred, and the 15 people listed below—who are in a single atom-bomb shelter—are the only humans left alive on the earth. It will take two weeks for external radiation to drop to a safe survival level. Supplies in the shelter can just barely support seven people for two weeks;

the rest must be turned out to die so that those seven can survive. You, and the other members of your group, must decide who the survivors will be—and the group decision must be unanimous.

1. *Dr. Dane:* 39, no religious affiliation, Ph.D. in history, college professor, good health, married (one child, Bobby), active in community, white.

2. *Mrs. Dane:* 38, Jew, AB and MA in Psychology, counselor in mental health clinic, good health, married (one child, Bobby), active in community, white.

3. *Bobby Dane:* 10, Jew, special education classes for four years, mentally retarded (IQ 70), good health, enjoys his pets, white.

4. *Mrs. Garcia:* 33, Spanish-American, Roman Catholic, 9th grade education, cocktail waitress, prostitute, good health, married at 16, divorced at 18, abandoned as a child, in foster home as a youth, attacked by foster father at age 12, ran away from home, returned to reformatory, stayed till 16 (one child, three weeks old, Jean).

5. *Jean Garcia:* Three weeks old, Spanish-American, good health, nursing for food.

6. *Mrs. Evans:* 30, negro, Protestant, AB and MA in elementary education, teacher, divorced (one child, Mary), in good health, cited as outstanding teacher, enjoys working with children.

7. *Mary Evans:* 8, negro, Protestant, 3rd grade, good health, excellent student.

8. *John Jacobs:* 13, white, Protestant, 6th grade, good health, excellent student.

9. *Mr. Newton:* 25, negro, claims to be an atheist, starting last year of medical school, suspended, homosexual activity, good health, seems bitter concerning racial problems, wears hippy clothes.

10. *Sister Mary Kathleen:* 27, nun, college graduate, English major, grew up in upper middle-class neighborhood, good health, her father was a businessman.

11. *Mr. Clark:* 28, negro, college graduate, BS in electronics engineering, married (no children), good health, enjoys outdoor sports and stereo equipment, grew up in a ghetto.

12. *Mr. Blake:* 31, white, Mormon, BS graduate, mechanic, Mr. Fix-it, married (four children, not with him), good health, enjoys outdoors and working in his shop.

13. *Miss Allen:* 21, Spanish-American, Protestant, college senior, majored in nursing, good health, enjoys outdoor sports, likes people.

14. *Fr. Evans:* 37, white, Catholic priest, college plus seminary, active in civil rights, criticized for liberal views, good health, former college athlete.

15. *Dr. Gonzales:* 66, Spanish-American, Catholic, MD, general practitioner, has had two heart attacks in past five years but continues to practice.

The teacher can conduct a discussion with the total class, at which time each group can report the reasoning behind its choices. During such a discussion, emphasis should be placed upon why certain people were chosen over others. Groups which disagree should be encouraged to be accepting of others' values and not feel compelled to encourage others to agree with their choices.

Value Judgment

Like the exercise just described, Value Judgment ranks people in order to investigate the worth attributed to particular behaviors. Again the class is divided into groups of six students each, and a handout containing the following information—and Fig. 3.3—is given to each student:

> There are two islands close together in the ocean, but because of sharks in the water it is impossible to cross from one to the other without a boat. On West Island there are one woman (X), two men $(A$ and $B)$, and a boat. On East Island there are two men $(C$ and $D)$, but no boat. X is in love with C and wants to go to him, but she doesn't know how to handle the boat. She asks A to take her to East Island, but he does not want to hear about her problems or become involved in them. He wants to be left alone.
>
> B offers to take X to East Island, but only if she spends the night with him first. She agrees. Next day, after X has gotten over to East Island, C dis-

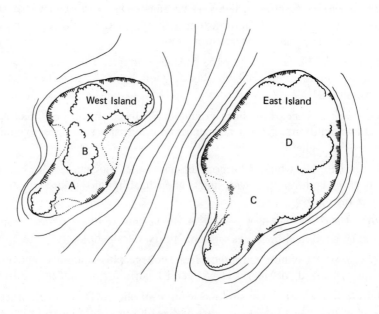

Figure 3.3

covers the circumstances under which she got there, and wants nothing more to do with her.

D, on the other hand, doesn't care what she's done or why. He'll take her under any circumstances.

Your task is to rank these people in order from the one you respect most to the one you respect least.

A discussion of each group's rankings will elicit conclusions similar to those of the Who Should Survive? activity.

Proud Statement

Everyone has something of which to be proud. Often, however, people never stop to think of how proud they should be and at what specifics their pride should be directed. The time taken in class to ask students to verbally complete the statement, "I am proud that I . . ." is time well spent. The appeal to positive traits has long been recognized as worthwhile in the educational setting.[3] The Proud Statement exercise is just one method in which to use the positive nature of students. When the rationale for each proud statement is discussed by the student making the statement, it often evokes very heart-warming feelings in the listeners. The students usually become more thoughtful and appreciative of their own worth and the value of their classmates as a result of this exercise.

Fantasy Questions

When students are confronted with open-ended questions calling for imagination, their answers are often indicative of their values. Some examples of such questions follow:

1. If you were a color, what color would you like to be?
2. If you were a food, what food would you like to be?
3. In which period in history would you have liked to live?
4. If you were a piece of furniture, which piece of furniture would you like to be?
5. If you were a flower, which flower would you like to be?
6. If you were an animal, which animal would you like to be?
7. If you could perform one miracle, what would that miracle be?
8. If you had a million dollars, what would be the first thing that you would buy?
9. During next weekend what would you like to do?
10. If you were a television program, what program would you like to be?
11. If you were a day of the week, what day would you like to be?

12. If you were an electric appliance, which one would you like to be?

13. If you were a parent, what would you like to do with your children?

14. If you were a smell, what smell would you like to be?

15. If you were a part of a body, what part would you like to be?

A discussion of these responses in small groups is recommended. Since no answers are either wrong or right, students should be instructed to ask questions of each other which will help to clarify why they responded as they did; rather than to persuade one another that their responses were most creative.

Epitaph

The purpose of having students deal with values choices is perhaps best served by confronting them with the purpose of their very existence. This exercise requires students to imagine their own deaths and compose their own epitaphs. In this manner they decide what they would like to be able to say about themselves at the conclusion of life. In other words, the question for each student becomes: What do I want my life to have meant?" When the epitaphs have been written, and the discussion turns to how the students can best deserve the epitaphs they have written for themselves, the result will be that each student will have devised means of being what he or she wants to become.

Similarly, students can be asked to write their own obituaries.

Making Lists

The development of lists can help clarify values and help people behave consistently with the values they profess. For example, the students can be asked to develop a list of things that would make them feel good. Next, they list obstacles to achieving those things, and the resources and strategies they can employ to overcome these obstacles.

Likewise, students can list those things they have to do—then ways of feeling better about these things (perhaps by combining them with activities they enjoy).

The possible listings are limited only by the health teacher's creativity and ingenuity.

Values Check

A grid can be handed out to periodically check one's values. Utilizing the three aspects of value clarification processing, the grid takes the form shown on the following page. The numbered columns at the right coincide with the seven questions at the bottom of the grid. The student's task is to check those boxes representing the criteria (the seven questions) that he or she has met. A sub-

Stated Issue	1	2	3	4	5	6	7
I favor rational decisions.							
I am opposed to abortion.							
I care about people.							
Etc.							

1. Are you *proud* of (do you prize or cherish) your position?
2. Have you *publicly affirmed* your position?
3. Have you chosen your position from *alternatives?*
4. Have you chosen your position after *thoughtful consideration?*
5. Have you chosen your position *freely?*
6. Have you *acted* consistently with your position?
7. Have you acted with *repetition or consistency* on this issue?

sequent task becomes an attempt to meet those criteria for which the student has not previously accounted. The development of strategies to account for the unmet criteria should then be commenced.

-ly Descriptions

On a two-foot square sheet of oak tag paper, students can be requested to list, using large letters, five descriptions of how they think they act. These descriptions must end in the letters "ly"; e.g., cruelly, sweetly, crazily, interestingly, etc. A piece of yarn can be placed through two holes—one at each top corner—so that the oak tag sheet with the five descriptions can be worn around the neck, like an "Eat at Joe's" sign. Then the students are requested to walk around the classroom and nonverbally show agreement or disagreement with others' descriptions of their behavior. For instance, after stopping to read student A's descriptions, student B might point to one of these descriptions and shake his head vigorously yes or no to indicate strong agreement or disagreement with it. This phase of the -ly descriptions exercise gives students the opportunity to receive feedback from their peers about their behavior, as well as a chance to engage in some introspection of their behavior.

The second phase of this exercise requires students to trade one or more of their five descriptions to another student for one or more of that student's descriptions. So that, for example, student A might trade a "cruelly" for student B's "belligerently." In this manner, students inspect their values pertaining to these behaviors and must judge some to be more worthwhile than others. Obviously student A, in the example just cited, values "belligerently" more than "cruelly," since he was willing to part with "cruelly" and substitute "belligerently."

The last phase of this activity is conducted in small groups where the rationale for each trade is presented by the traders.

Role Trading

Somewhat like -ly Descriptions, this activity calls for students to place a role that they play on an index card. Each student writes six roles for himself or herself—one per index card—so that he or she has six index cards. Possible roles are: brother, sister, student, friend, athlete, etc. When all have written their cards, the students walk around the room and, nonverbally, give to some other students the three roles that they *least value*.

A small or large group discussion should then relate to the following questions:

1. How would you feel about giving away these three roles if you *really* had to do that?
2. How would you feel about *really* accepting the roles others gave you?
3. How important to you are the three roles you were unwilling to give away?
4. How well do you perform the roles you valued most?
5. How could you perform better the roles you valued most?

Learning Statements

Since the school setting is one in which learning is expected to occur, and since the purpose of values clarification is related to an introspection and cognizance of one's values, students should periodically be asked to write a couple of sentences, paragraphs, or pages beginning with the phrase, "I learned that I . . . ." Participation in values clarification activities is very valuable for understanding one's values, but the additional task of specifying what one has learned about oneself adds considerably to the worth of these exercises.

After conducting values clarification exercises with a heterogeneous group of teachers and students in a workshop setting, Learning Statements were submitted to this author. It seems appropriate to end this section with some of those statements:

I learned that I am one hell of a lot better off than I thought I was.

I learned that I can communicate with older people quite easily when I want to, that we can learn to live together in society, that I can respect their views if they respect mine.

I learned that I find young people fun, interesting, and concerned.

TO FOLLOW

The following chapters are divided by health content study areas and are meant to employ the knowledge, attitudes, and skills developed through group process and values clarification activities. Since valuing is such an integral correlate to health behavior, activities are provided to explore values related to each of the content areas. Likewise, activities of a small- and large-group nature are interspersed throughout. In all cases, however, the activities involve the active participation of students in the learning process.

REFERENCES

1. Louis Raths, Merrill Harmin, and Sidney Simon, *Values and Teaching: Working with Values in the Classroom* (Columbus, Ohio: Charles E. Merrill, 1966).
2. A more detailed explanation of the theory behind the values clarification technique can be acquired from Raths et al.
3. Portia E. Perry, "Behavior Modification and Social Learning Theory: Application in the School," *Journal of Education* **53,** 4 (1971), p. 20.

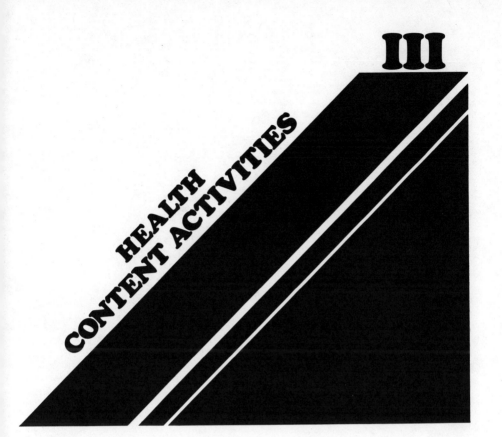

HEALTH
CONTENT ACTIVITIES

III

Instructional Strategies for Mental Health

The title of this chapter refers to a state of well-being. Some excellent mental health education programs are being conducted by health instructors. Unfortunately, some other programs are preoccupied with mental *illness* as opposed to mental *health*. Since educators are not prepared for the role of therapist, deep-seated psychological disturbances characteristic of some children can not adequately be responded to by the health teacher. In cases of this type, the health teacher's responsibility is to refer such students to those who are better able to help them. To be sure, an understanding of mental illnesses is worthwhile. However, the view expressed in this chapter will be one of prevention and exploration. Feelings of alienation and self-depreciation will be prevented; one's feelings toward oneself and others will be explored, as well as the means of bettering one's mental health status and decreasing loneliness and isolation.

INTRODUCTORY ACTIVITIES

This section concerns itself with instructional strategies to increase trust in the classroom, while at the same time providing the opportunity for introspective deliberations.

"Tell Me"

The "Tell me" game can be organized to be played in pairs or small groups from four to six students. The object of this exercise is to help students get to know one another better and feel more comfortable with one another. In order for these objectives to be met, statements beginning with "Tell me" are developed and responded to by the participants. Though students once familiar with the exercise can develop their own "Tell me" statements, it is recommended that initially the teacher create them. Once a number of such statements are developed, each student chooses one to ask another student. Should a youngster who was not asked to respond to a particular "Tell me" desire to, he or she should be allowed that opportunity. Pupils should be cautioned to react honestly and in some detail to these statements for the objectives of this exercise to be best served. Examples of "Tell me" statements are:

1. Tell me something about your family.
2. Tell me something that you like about yourself.
3. Tell me something that you dislike about yourself.
4. Tell me what you like and dislike about school.
5. Tell me which parts of your body you like least and which parts you like best.

6. Tell me your most vivid elementary school memory.
7. Tell me about the best thing that ever happened to you.
8. Tell me a secret.
9. Tell me how you feel about this class.
10. Tell me what you enjoy doing.
11. Tell me about a turning point in your life.
12. Tell me about your greatest success.
13. Tell me about your greatest failure.
14. Tell me what you would like to do after you are finished with your schooling.
15. Tell me about the person who has most influenced you in your life.
16. Tell me how you feel about dying.
17. Tell me what you like to eat.
18. Tell me what you look for in a friend.
19. Tell me what you fear.
20. Tell me what you think of yourself.

Conversation Starters

Similar in purpose to the "Tell me" game, this exercise utilizes incomplete sentences rather than "Tell me" statements. The following conversation starters were distributed in a workshop session conducted by Bill Blokker at State University of New York at Buffalo in 1973.

1. Other people usually . . .
2. The best measure of personal success is . . .
3. Anybody will work hard if . . .
4. People will think of me as . . .
5. When I let go . . . .
6. Marriage can be . . .
7. Nothing is so frustrating as . . .
8. People who run things should be . . .
9. I miss . . .
10. The thing I like about myself is . . .
11. There are times when I . . .
12. I would like to be . . .
13. When I have something to say . . .
14. As a child I . . .

15. The teacher I liked best was a person who . . .
16. It is fun to . . .
17. My body is . . .
18. When it comes to girls . . .
19. Loving someone . . .
20. Ten years from now, I . . .

Once the class becomes more trusting of one another, more intimate sentence completions can be discussed. Some possibilities are:

1. In the bathroom . . .
2. I used to daydream that . . .
3. At night I . . .
4. When I first heard a profane word I . . .
5. When I first saw a naked person I . . .
6. My religion is . . .
7. I feel most ashamed about . . .
8. I'm turned on by . . .
9. Right now I'm most reluctant to discuss . . .
10. I feel that you . . .
11. The thing I dislike most about this group is . . .
12. Girls (boys) think I . . .
13. I need . . .
14. My body . . .
15. The first chance I get, I'll . . .

"You're Like"

Rather than having one student reveal something about him- or herself to others, this activity requires others to reveal their perceptions of the one student they are focusing upon. In small groups of five students, four students give their responses to statements which refer to the fifth. Each pupil in turn has his or her chance to be focused upon. Examples of "You're Like" statements are:

1. Your childhood . . .
2. You get angry at . . .
3. You enjoy . . .
4. You care deeply about . . .
5. You will . . .

6. You think this school . . .
7. You would like to be . . .
8. You would like the teacher to . . .
9. You would like us as group members to . . .
10. The thing you dislike most about yourself is . . .
11. The thing you like most about yourself is . . .
12. You like people who . . .
13. People don't like you when . . .
14. You feel hurt when . . .
15. You really are . . .
16. In front of boys (girls) you feel . . .
17. When you lose a game you . . .
18. When you're alone you . . .
19. You feel like smiling when . . .
20. Right now you feel . . .

Perceptions Survey

Another means of aiding students to see themselves as others see them is through use of the survey technique. Having organized the students into groups of six, the teacher hands out the following Perceptions Survey:

Perceptions survey

Directions: Fill in the name of the person in your group, other than yourself, who you think *best* fits the descriptions below. Place that name on the line to the left of the description. Each description *must* have one, and only one, name associated with it, but the same person's name can be used to answer more than one question. Do not discuss your answers with anyone in the group until the teacher requests you to.

_____ 1. Who is the kindest?
_____ 2. Who is the cruelest?
_____ 3. Who is likely to do anonymous favors for people?
_____ 4. Who is afraid of mice?
_____ 5. Who cheats on exams?
_____ 6. Who is careless?
_____ 7. Who is very careful?
_____ 8. Who enjoys music?

_____ 9. Who enjoys sports?

_____ 10. Who wears seat belts?

_____ 11. Who likes chocolate layer cakes?

_____ 12. Who rarely has a cavity?

_____ 13. Who dislikes school?

_____ 14. Who butters up the teacher?

_____ 15. Who wakes up often with nightmares?

_____ 16. Who will make a good parent?

_____ 17. Who is a good child?

_____ 18. Who is most materialistic?

_____ 19. Who enjoys danger?

_____ 20. Who would be a good teacher?

_____ 21. Who would be a good friend?

_____ 22. Who likes pets?

_____ 23. Who might use drugs?

_____ 24. Who is afraid of being alone?

_____ 25. Who would like to be someone other than who he or she is?

_____ 26. Who cares a lot about his or her reputation?

_____ 27. Who enjoys classical music?

_____ 28. Who feels most sad?

_____ 29. Who is most happy?

_____ 30. Who has the most secrets?

_____ 31. Who doesn't sleep enough?

_____ 32. Who feels most comfortable with his or her body?

_____ 33. Who needs something?

_____ 34. In twenty years who will most likely smoke cigarettes?

_____ 35. In twenty years, who will most likely be unhealthy?

_____ 36. Who would make a good judge?

_____ 37. Who would make a good scientist?

_____ 38. Who would make a good guidance counselor?

_____ 39. Who is most serious?

_____ 40. Who will be most religious?

_____41. Who will be most popular?

_____42. Who will spank his or her children?

_____43. Who will choose not to marry?

_____44. Who reads the most?

_____45. Who reads the least?

_____46. Who daydreams the most?

_____47. Who has enjoyed filling out this questionnaire the least?

_____48. Who has enjoyed filling out this questionnaire the most?

_____49. Who is most likely to become a television personality?

_____50. Who would want to change his or her name?

When all the students have completed the survey, they are asked to write each group member's name on a separate sheet of paper, then to place the *number* of each description under the *name* they associated with that description. The results of this procedure might appear as:

John	Harry	Beth
2,6,23,33	1,3,7,16,22	14,20,27,44,48

The next step requires the students to discuss the results of this survey in their groups by focusing on one student at a time. In this manner, each student will have insight into how five classmates perceive him or her and his or her behavior. Generalizations should be drawn from each set of perceptions. For example, the results cited above might lead to the following generalizations:

1. John needs help to change. If that help doesn't come, he might one day abuse drugs or turn to some other deviant behavior.

2. Harry interacts well with others. He is well liked and will therefore relate well with other people regardless of the situation.

3. Beth is very smart. She will do best at those things requiring thought and logic. Her enjoyment will probably not be derived from other people but rather from things (books, classical music, questionnaires, etc.).

There are those who would object to negative perceptions and generalizations such as those concerning John. These teachers could change the negative descriptions in the survey to positive statements. However, the value of this exercise might then be subverted. If the objective is to afford students the opportunity to see themselves through others' eyes, they must be allowed to receive —and should expect—honest responses. The attitude that ignorance is bliss, and that therefore a student perceived by others in a negative manner should not be made aware of these perceptions, is one that will not help students to grow and develop in a socially functional manner. The first step to becoming a better person is to find out the kind of person one is. Exploration of the perceptions others have of one is a necessary ingredient for the improvement of oneself. Of course, the teacher and students should understand and agree with this posture or else this activity might be dysfunctional. Some teachers and some students may not be ready for such honesty.

Perceptual Set

A logical follow-up to the perceptual survey is an exercise which will demonstrate the importance of how others perceive us in relation to how they treat and receive us. The teacher arranges for a speaker to visit the school one day and talk about some controversial topic; e.g., some aspect of sexual behavior. The speaker is told to give a "neutral" speech; i.e., to neither advocate nor reject the sexual behavior about which he or she is talking. Three different health education classes, preferably similar to one another in terms of student intelligence, age, etc., are prepared for the speaker in different ways. One class is offered a positive perceptual set of the speaker by being given and asked to read the following biographical data sheet at the beginning of the class period in which the guest will talk to the class:

> Bob Jones is a young activist who has worked continually for sexual freedom for students like yourselves. He has even been arrested and locked in jail when he interfered with the police as they were hassling a young girl outside a local high school. The young girl was being bothered by the police for not having worn a brassiere to school. Bob often talks with young people about sex and has just turned down a job paying much more than he presently makes just so he can continue to meet with young people as he is today. I'm sure that you'll enjoy Bob's stay with us.

The second class is offered a neutral perceptual set of the speaker and his visit:

> Robert Jones is a man who speaks to people about sexuality. Mr. Jones will talk for fifteen to twenty minutes today about this topic. I now present Mr. Robert Jones.

The third class is presented a negative perceptual set for the presentation:

> Robert Jones is a speaker who has the reputation of often distorting the truth. He is regarded as only interested in himself and his own sexual hang-ups. Mr. Jones' experiences have led many schools to prohibit his speaking to students, since students have always been appalled at his lack of knowledge and disregard for young people.

Let me just add that I would prefer not having to introduce Mr. Jones in this way, but I want you to view his presentation very critically and not be taken in by his act. I now present, quite reluctantly, Mr. Robert Jones.

No questions are allowed after the presentation (15–20 minutes) is finished. Instead, the students are asked to complete the following questionnaire:

SPEAKER REACTION FORM
Health Education Class

Name _____ Period_____

Directions

On the basis of your impressions of this person, check *one* alternative in each set which you feel would most accurately describe him. Work quickly, and check the alternative that most closely matches your impression.

1. In general, how does he get along with other people?
____ a. Very well, with friends, but only if he knows them well.
____ b. People are impressed until they really get to know him.
____ c. Is well liked, meets people easily.
____ d. Is respected rather than liked.

2. What does his attitude toward others seem to be?
____ a. Cold and distant.
____ b. Somewhat indifferent to others.
____ c. Really likes others, enjoys meeting them.
____ d. Tends to take advantage of people, uses people.

3. How responsive to people is he?
____ a. Often reserved and aloof, somewhat distant.
____ b. Very warm and open with almost everyone.
____ c. A little distrustful of people, always on guard.
____ d. Attempts to be "warm," but really isn't.

4. How would his temperament best be described?
____ a. Somewhat excitable and emotional.
____ b. Serious, cautious.
____ c. Cool, calculating.
____ d. Tends to be a stable person, calm, easy-going.

5. How might he behave in an argument?
____ a. Remains calm, reasonable, and controlled.
____ b. Agrees on the surface, but is quite rigid.
____ c. May side with other's point of view to avoid a scene.
____ d. Becomes angry, belligerent.

6. How would he react to criticism?

_____ a. Shows resentment.
_____ b. Ignores it.
_____ c. Outwardly accepts it, but inwardly seeks revenge.
_____ d. Is hurt, very sensitive, but keeps it to himself.

7. How does he feel about students?

_____ a. Sincerely likes them and shows it.
_____ b. Admires them but resents and envies them.
_____ c. Is tolerant of their beliefs.
_____ d. Appears to like them, but really thinks he is better than they are.

8. What is his greatest strength?

_____ a. Loyalty, trustworthiness.
_____ b. Sense of humor, keen wit.
_____ c. Intelligence.
_____ d. Shrewdness.

9. What is his primary life goal?

_____ a. To have enough security and be comfortable.
_____ b. To help others (e.g., the poor, the ill), to be a "good samaritan."
_____ c. Success and recognition.
_____ d. To receive high esteem from others.

10. What about himself is he most proud of?

_____ a. Intelligence.
_____ b. Ability to understand people.
_____ c. Sincerity, honesty.
_____ d. Ability to manipulate people.

11. What is his real opinion of sex education?

_____ a. Sincerely believes in it.
_____ b. Acts interested but is really indifferent.
_____ c. Actively supports it.
_____ d. Tolerates it but is doubtful as to its effectiveness.

Go on to the following exercise:

Directions

Check one adjective or phrase in each pair which best describes the person you have just heard.

1. _____ a. concerned with self 3. _____ a. sincere
   _____ b. concerned with others   _____ b. phony

2. _____ a. sense of humor 4. _____ a. suspicious
   _____ b. stern, business-like   _____ b. trusting

5. ___ a. vindictive
   ___ b. forgiving
6. ___ a. dependable
   ___ b. undependable
7. ___ a. progressive
   ___ b. conservative
8. ___ a. scheming
   ___ b. humble
9. ___ a. honest
   ___ b. two-faced
10. ___ a. condescending
    ___ b. considerate
11. ___ a. tolerant
    ___ b. prejudiced
12. ___ a. conscientious
    ___ b. self-centered

13. ___ a. intelligent
    ___ b. shrewd
14. ___ a. optimistic
    ___ b. realistic
15. ___ a. honest
    ___ b. untrustworthy
16. ___ a. kind
    ___ b. inconsiderate
17. ___ a. opinionated, dogmatic
    ___ b. flexible, open
18. ___ a. warm, friendly
    ___ b. cold, indifferent
19. ___ a. selfish
    ___ b. generous
20. Would you like to get to know
    him better?
    ___ a. Yes
    ___ b. No

Prior to the next meeting of these three health education classes, the teacher should tabulate the results of the questionnaire and ditto these so that a copy may be distributed to each student. The results should be tabulated by class (actually perceptual set) and the responses of all three classes to the questionnaire should be distributed to each student. Invariably there will be a difference in the results between that class which received the positive perceptual set and that class which received the negative perceptual set.

The teacher then lets the classes in on the "secret," and discussions pertaining to the importance of people's perceptions of others are conducted. It is worthwhile for the teacher to mention that people behave in terms of their *perceptions* of reality, and not necessarily in terms of what *is* reality. Through this procedure, the perceptions of themselves gleaned through the Perceptual Survey exercise take on added significance for these students.

FEELINGS ACTIVITIES

The reader is now asked to list three feelings he or she has about this book. Please do not read further until this is done.

Was your list similar to the following?

1. I think this book is great.
2. The author is unrealistic.
3. Some of these activities are tremendous.

4. The book is too short (long).

5. I wish this book were available much earlier.

Or did your list include items such as these?

1. I feel frustrated that I can't teach this way.

2. I feel confused.

3. I feel enthusiastic and want to try some of these activities.

4. I feel close to the author.

5. I feel a sense of worthiness since I've been doing exercises like these with my classes before I ever read the book.

It must be obvious now that the first set of statements above are thoughts, beliefs, or opinions—but not *feelings*. The second set of statements expresses the feelings of frustration, confusion, enthusiasm, psychological closeness, and self-worth. If you found that the three feelings you liked about this book were everything but feelings, do not fret. Most respondents would exhibit the same behavior, since we are not used to identifying our feelings, or writing or speaking about them. In fact, we are quite talented in hiding the feelings we have. As a means of practicing feeling responses, why not mail to this author your feelings as you read this book?

This section will be devoted to instructional methodologies designed to aid students in developing the ability to recognize the feelings of themselves and others and to respond appropriately to those feelings which are identified. As the first suggestion in this section, it is recommended the teacher conduct the same activity as employed by the author to introduce feelings. The teacher's question might be: "How do you feel during health education class?" The following activities will be based on the assumption that this suggestion has been taken, and now the students know how feeling responses differ from thoughts, beliefs, and opinions.

Acting Out Feelings

Emotional health and the study of feelings is one of the more difficult topics to investigate in a school setting. One exercise which is valuable in helping students understand their feelings and emotions in an interesting manner is to act out various feelings. Students are either asked to volunteer to act out one of the feelings in the following list, or they may be assigned a feeling to role-play. Role-playing may be limited to verbal expressions only, physical movements only, or a combination of both. Discussions of the acting and the feeling are included as a part of this exercise. Feelings which may be role-played are:

1. pride	5. love	9. freedom
2. happiness	6. sadness	10. fascination
3. glory	7. joy	11. loneliness
4. determination	8. warmth	12. confidence

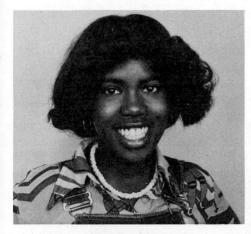

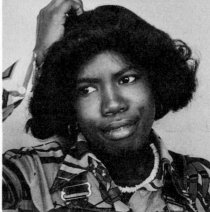

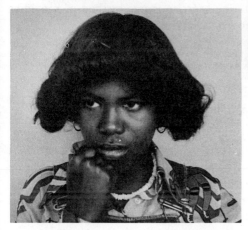

This student is Acting Out Feelings. First happy, next contemplative, and lastly angry.

After a student acts out a feeling, the rest of the students in the group must attempt to guess what that feeling was. If they are unable to, the actor must role-play another feeling. An analysis of why the group could not guess the feeling being portrayed will be helpful to subsequent role-players.

If conducted nonverbally, this exercise highlights the relationship of body position to emotional set. For example, a happy, joyous feeling might result in a straight-backed, tall, bouncy body position; whereas a feeling of sadness might be manifested physically by a stance with shoulders rounded, head down, arms drooping. The realization that the body position often indicates feelings, is one which will help students to identify what others are feeling at times when those others are not communicating their feelings verbally.

Staring

The class is divided into groups of six students each. One of the six volunteers to be "it" and stands, while the remaining five students also stand and form a circle around "it." The teacher directs those in the circle to stare at the student in the center of the circle. They are to do nothing else; i.e., they may not talk or make any attempt at nonverbal communication. The staring should continue for three minutes.

Though these three minutes will seem like an eternity, the behavior manifested by "it" will allow for a meaningful discussion of feelings at the conclusion of this exercise. Such behavior as fidgeting, nervous laughter, swaying, making funny faces at the other students, looking up, or looking down will be evidence of feeling responses. If videotape equipment is available, these behaviors can be captured on tape to be replayed, as the students who were on the outside of the circle guess how "it" feels from the behavior he or she shows. "It" should attempt to recall how he or she felt at that particular moment, so as to verify or correct the group's guess about his or her feelings.

It is necessary for the health educator to remember that skills such as being able to detect feelings in oneself and others do not just develop. They take a lot of practice, as do other skills. The staring exercise is one method of providing this practice in a manner which is interesting and educational.

Break in the Circle

Most people have been excluded from some group at sometime—whether from a country club because of religion, a community because of race, a social group because of values, a sports team for lack of ability. Not surprisingly, the feeling of rejection is intense. To demonstrate rejection from a group, have 10 students form a circle, all facing the center. These students represent a group who wants no part of another student who is on the outside of the circle; it's the in-group versus the outsider. Members of the in-group interlock hands or arms and must not allow the outsider to enter the circle (group). The outsider's task is to get into the circle—first by coercion and verbally requesting entry, then by physically breaking into the circle. The participants should be forewarned not to engage in any dangerous behavior such as punching, pinching, or any other means of breaking the circle which might result in injury to a player.

There are several methods of analyzing this activity at its conclusion. The insiders and the outsiders should try to clarify for each other how they felt. If the group is effective in preventing entry, frustration and rejection are usually experienced by the outsider; whereas the other participants feel camaraderie, joy, and success. If the outsider does break through the circle, it should be observed whether he or she enters the center of the circle (still distinct from the rest of the players) or attempts to hold hands or interlock arms with the insiders (to be one of the group). In any case, students should be aware of their feelings during all phases of this exercise.

A variation of the format described above, is for the students in the circle to face outward from the center. This indicates a conscious effort to keep out the "intruder," while facing in could connote an attitude of ignoring the outsider.

It would be useful to compare these two methods, facing in and facing out, in relation to the feelings they evoke in the participants.

Shouting Names

Malamud and Machover[1] describe a game whose function is to put people in touch with their feelings. To conduct this activity, the teacher asks for several volunteers. Then the teacher selects one of these volunteers at a time and instructs the remainder of the class to shout, in unison, the name of that volunteer. The name is shouted three times. When all the volunteers have had their names shouted three times by the class, a discussion is conducted of the feelings of both the volunteers and the shouters. Some volunteers find that they enjoy the attention while others do not. The authors report one student volunteer wincing as if being scolded, while another smiled from ear to ear, indicating the pleasure he was feeling. Relative to the shouters, some enjoy the freedom to "let go" a tremendous shout, while others feel self-conscious. Malamud and Machover report feelings of inadequacy and self-consciousness, and needs for exhibitionism evidenced on the part of the shouters.

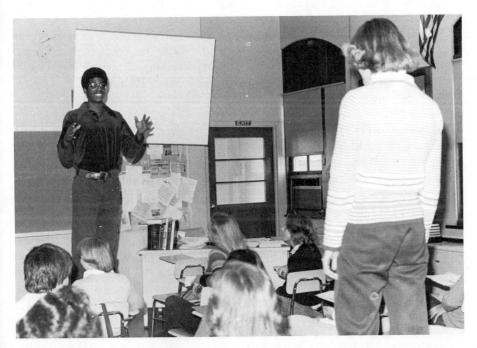

These students are participating in the Shouting Names activity. This instructional strategy can be an excellent manner of introducing a discussion on feelings.

Gracious Receiving

One of the more difficult tasks for people is to receive compliments in an accepting fashion. Upon being complimented, some people make strange comments and/or show strange feelings. For example:

Compliment: My, what a nice hat you're wearing.
Response: Oh, it's not new anymore.

Compliment: I felt like getting you this gift.
Response: Oh, you shouldn't have.

Compliment: My, you look pretty today.
Response: You probably say that to all the girls.

Compliment: You know, you're a real nice person.
Response: Oh, go on.

The next activity is designed to have students identify and analyze the feelings they experience when they're being complimented. The class is divided into groups of six students each, and each group member gets a turn to be the focus of the group's compliments. The compliments must be truthful.

The task of the participants is to attempt to understand their feelings both while they are being complimented and when they are doing the complimenting. A discussion held at the conclusion of this exercise should focus upon these feelings as well as on how best to respond to compliments.

A variation of this procedure calls for "it" to tell the group a thing of which he or she is proud. The other participants continually interrupt to compliment "it" on those parts of his or her story that are deserving of compliment. A discussion, similar to the one described above, then ends this exercise.

The outcomes of Gracious Receiving are students' realizations that receiving and expressing positive feelings can be nice; that inhibiting expression of these feelings deprives both the giver and the receiver of this niceness; and that expression of positive feelings brings people closer to each other. These are indeed important lessons to be learned.

Blocking

It is often difficult for people to identify with those different from themselves. Blocking is a game which can be employed to develop empathy for others. The health educator should request the shop teacher to supply him or her with enough two-inch by two-inch wooden blocks for each student in the class. The instructor then distributes these blocks to the class, requesting that each student carry the block from that moment until the same time the next day (24 hours). The block is *never* to leave the hand except when the students are sleeping. They will have to hold the block while eating, showering, playing sports, etc.

At the next meeting of that health education class, the teacher should discuss with the students their experiences and feelings related to carrying the block. Some students will have felt self-conscious, others ridiculous, and still others burdened. The teacher then draws an analogy between the block and some burdens that people carry with them all the time. For example, fat is the obese person's block; pimples are the blocks for people with acne. The feelings of self-consciousness, ridiculousness, and being burdened that the students felt for a short period of time, are often felt by people with different "blocks" *all* the time. That some people make fun of others different from themselves, thereby making their "blocks" even heavier to carry, should be discussed.

Friends and Enemies

To aid students to experience and investigate a wide range of feelings, have them think of one friend and one enemy. On one sheet of paper they should list five adjectives that they think their friend would use to support them; on another sheet of paper they should list five adjectives describing themselves which their enemy might use to tear them down. These adjectives should be words which actually are, or have been, used by others to describe these students. The class is then organized into pairs to discuss the feelings evoked when the supporting adjectives are used by the friend and the downgrading adjectives are used by the enemy—*and* what would be felt if the friend used the negative adjectives and the enemy the positive ones in a description of that student. Is it the word, the person who uses the word, or a combination of the two which most affects the feeling response.

How/When Questionnaire

One device with which to help students identify how they feel during various occasions is the How/When questionnaire. Students are asked to identify *how* they feel *when* something happens. The questionnaire should be completed individually and then discussed in pairs or small groups. Discussion should relate to why such feelings are experienced at those particular times. Some How/When items might be:

_____ 1. How do you feel when you fail a test in school?

_____ 2. How do you feel when you lose a game?

_____ 3. How do you feel when you get turned down for a date?

_____ 4. How do you feel when you're called to answer a question in class?

_____ 5. How do you feel when you get punished?

_____ 6. How do you feel when you are complimented?

_____ 7. How do you feel when you get a bad haircut?

_____ 8. How do you feel when you disappoint your parents?

_____ 9. How do you feel when it rains?

_____10. How do you feel when it snows?

_____11. How do you feel when the sun shines?

_____12. How do you feel when you cheat at something?

_____13. How do you feel when you have a big problem?

_____14. How do you feel when you've won a prize?

_____15. How do you feel when you get selected?

_____16. How do you feel when you are with your best friend?

_____17. How do you feel when you get hurt?

_____18. How do you feel when you go to the dentist?

_____19. How do you feel when winter comes?

_____20. How do you feel when you come to school?

Student responses should be placed on the line to the left of the item to which that response relates.

Feeling Drawings

Feelings may be expressed by colors (red for active and pale blue for passive, for instance) or through drawings. This activity requires students to depict their feelings in a drawing. They might be asked to draw their feelings about:

1. competition
2. winning
3. losing
4. surprising
5. loving
6. caring
7. cooperating
8. sharing
9. learning
10. parenting

The artists then display their drawings and briefly report to the class what they drew and why they drew it the way they did.

Self-Incorporated

An interesting use of instructional materials is to present situations that can elicit discussions of feelings which might otherwise not be possible. Films used in such a manner are called "trigger films," since they employ on-screen events to trigger discussion. It is felt that an analysis of the on-screen events will initially be less threatening to the students than discussions related to their own feelings. A skillful teacher, however, can facilitate the discussion in such a way as to move from the on-screen event to the students' own lives.

An excellent instructional material that can be used to trigger discussions with students in mental health units is entitled *Self-Incorporated*.[2] Developed by a consortium of educational and broadcasting agencies, and an offshoot of the award winning *Inside/Outside* series, *Self-Incorporated* contains fifteen 15-minute color videotapes and/or films designed to help students cope with the emotional, physical, and social problems that confront them. The topics presented in the series include:

1. Skills needed to work for change within social systems
2. Coping with emotions related to physiological change
3. The need for individual and group membership
4. Societal ambiguity about male and female roles
5. Skills needed for dealing with family adversity
6. Coping with failure reasonably
7. Understanding the family and its members
8. Appreciating that feelings of anxiety about interacting with persons of the opposite sex are normal
9. Understanding the need for ethnic identity as well as the qualities common to all human beings
10. The need for privacy
11. Understanding and coping with pressure to succeed
12. Making self-enhancing decisions in the face of peer pressure
13. Dealing with being cast as good or bad
14. Recognizing and dealing with daily pressure
15. Making moral decisions

After viewing a tape or film, students can easily be brought to discuss topics with which they would not have felt comfortable previously. Small-group or large-group discussions are appropriate, with students being asked to describe instances in which they found themselves in circumstances similar to the characters just viewed.

ACTIVITIES TO AFFECT BEHAVIOR

This section includes activities designed to specifically relate to the ways in which students act, and means of behaving more consistently with their desires. Several of these exercises reflect the major concept of this book: as a popular song says: *people need people.* Therefore, students are organized to help other students meet their goals.

Prescriptions

During a visit with this author and his students, Dr. Gerald Edwards presented an exercise intended to result in suggested behaviors which students could adopt to feel less frustrated. The exercise required students to list those things they felt frustrated about on one side of a sheet of paper, and the way they felt about these frustrations on the other side of that paper. After trying several methods of processing this data, the students formed quartets to discuss their frustrations and feelings about them. Each quartet was asked to choose one member's frustrations to focus on, and to prescribe a specific behavior that person could follow for one week to attempt to relieve some of that frustration. The behavior prescribed had to be reasonable and of a type that could be expected to provide some measure of relief in a week's time. Each student in the quartet took a turn to be focused on.

Two particular means of prescribing these behaviors are recommended. The first approach calls for the student whose frustrations are being considered, to sit with his or her back to the other group members. The three other students then discuss that person's frustrations for three minutes, not allowing any verbalizing from the "focus." After three minutes of such discussion, in which specific behaviors are recommended, the "focus" reacts for one minute to what has been said.

The second method of prescribing behaviors requires each member to touch each other member of the quartet, one at a time (shake hands, place hand on shoulder or arm, etc.), and tell them, "This week I want you to. . . ." The physical contact is designed to create a feeling of closeness and concern on the part of the group's members.

Regardless of the method of prescribing behavior, time should be provided the next week for the quartets to reconvene and report to each other which behaviors they tried and the result of these attempts. The quartet might then want to suggest additional actions for its members to take.

A word about suggested behaviors: These should be specific. Suggestions such as "talk to someone" or "have fun" are not as meaningful as "talk to your parents about . . ." or "go to the school basketball game this Friday."

The results of this activity are severalfold:

1. Students come away with specific things they can do to overcome some of their frustrations.

2. A feeling that others care about them enough to want to help them relieve some frustration makes students feel less isolated.

3. Peer group pressure is utilized positively by being directed at making the group members feel better.

Telegramming

Though suggestions to help students achieve their goals are useful, often these suggestions are not adopted nor their goals accomplished. This activity is designed to remind students where they want to go (their goals) and how they can get there (suggested behaviors). Each pupil in the class is asked to send himself or herself a telegram specifying what he or she wants to accomplish in one month's time and what should be done to meet this end. The telegrams are written on sheets of paper which are then placed in envelopes distributed by the teacher, and the envelopes are sealed. The health instructor requests the students to address the envelopes to themselves and then collects them. In one month the teacher mails the envelopes to the students. After the students have received the envelopes, the class can, if desired, discuss the degree to which students have been successful in achieving their short-range goals. At this point, another telegram might be written which specifies a second goal, or, if the original goal has not been met, cites other behaviors which would aid in the achievement of that goal.

Permanent Grouping

Another means of aiding students to establish and move toward the satisfaction of short-range goals involves the establishment of small groups which meet every other week for one class period. These groups will be established for the life of the class to help their members develop rapport and caring for one another, and to allow for continuity in movement toward the goals cited by the group's members. At each meeting, once goals have been determined, the group should focus on identifying the forces present which seem to be assets in achieving the goals, and those which seem to be inhibiting their achievement. The task of the group then becomes one of developing strategies that members can employ to maximize the assets and minimize the inhibitors. Feedback on the effectiveness of these strategies should be a part of each group session. In this manner, the group serves as an ongoing advisory body concerned with the accomplishment of its members' goals. The phrase "all for one and one for all" comes to mind.

Justification of Self

For this exercise, the students are divided into groups of five. To bring students' past behavior into focus and to confront them with the meaning of that behavior, the following handout should be distributed to each group.

> An airplane on which you were flying to Europe from the United States, has crashed in the middle of the Atlantic Ocean and you are one of only five survivors. A life raft has been located, but it can only support three people without sinking. There is no possible way of switching people in and out, and, therefore, the *only* solution is to save three people in the raft and leave the other two behind. By describing your past deeds and explaining why they make you valuable to mankind, you must convince the other four people that you should be one of the three saved.

> Each of the five people in your group will make a three-minute presentation in an attempt to get into the life raft. After all the presentations have been

made, each person, in secret, will place on a sheet of paper the names of two other people in the group whom he or she wants to save. When this is done, count up the number of times each person's name appears on the sheets of paper. The three people whose names are most frequently mentioned are to be saved. If there is a tie for the third person, have the group vote between those who have tied.

This exercise requires students to consider the worth of their past behavior in relation to the needs of all men. Some students will conclude that they have been self-centered and have not functioned as contributing members of society. Other students will determine that they are proud of their concern for their fellow man, and will have their behavior reinforced.

SELF-CONCEPT ACTIVITIES

The activities included in this section are meant to help the students determine who they really are. They are designed to answer the existential question, "Who Am I?"

"I Am"

Since people in general seldom stop to think who or what they are, it is not surprising that students don't either. This exercise asks students to *list* as many characteristics of themselves as they can muster and that will fit on one-half of a sheet of paper (which does not include their name). The teacher collects these descriptions and tapes them on the walls of the classroom. The students are then told to walk around the room and write (in small letters, so as to leave room on the paper for others) the name of the person they think those characteristics describe. At the end of this phase of the exercise, the students are asked to take their own descriptions off the wall and determine who they were judged most often to be. Themselves? Someone else? If someone else, did they realize that they were perceived to be like this person? And as whom would they rather have been perceived?

Students will often find that their real self as perceived by others differs from the self *they* perceive. The question then becomes, "Who am I really?"

Self Portraits

A variation of the "I Am" game entails the drawing of one's self-portrait rather than the listing of characteristics. The portraits should be revealing, in some way, of the self the students perceive. As in the previous exercise, the portraits are taped to the walls and students wander about the room writing the name of the classmate they believe is being portrayed. A discussion of how the class' perceptions differ from the individual student's perceptions (or how they are similar) should include feelings elicited by and during this exercise.

Bravissimo

The purpose of this exercise is to help students learn more about themselves and others in their group in a positive experiential manner. In groups consisting of four students, each student in turn states—in only one sentence—something that he or she does, has done, or soon will do, about which he or she feels good. After each statement the group shouts "bravissimo," which means "very well done." After ten minutes of this activity, the groups should be allowed five minutes to have any of their members clarify a statement that has been made.

By allowing, and even requiring, students to focus on their positive behavior, and by having other students cheer this behavior, two main objectives are accomplished:

1. Students begin to realize, if they haven't before, that they have much of which to be proud.
2. Students' concepts of self are enhanced.

Fantasy Play

Many people desire to be someone other than who they are. The act of daydreaming about being someone else can be structured and used in fantasy plays. Students are organized into groups of six and then asked to imagine being someone other than themselves. The teacher should hasten to add that the someone else they are *imagining* should not be a real person, but rather an *imagined* one who possesses the personality, knowledge, skills, etc., that the student would like to possess. Each student then takes a turn to act out a one-minute play he or she developed which depicts this imaginary self. After each play, the other group members question the playwright to identify more clearly the traits of the imaginary self; then they suggest how the playwright might go about developing some of these characteristics. As stated elsewhere in this chapter, such suggestions should be realistic with some chance of succeeding.

This activity gives students a clearer concept of their real self, as well as concrete means for narrowing the gap between their ideal self and their real self.

VALUING ACTIVITIES

Values clarification can be employed to explore aspects of mental health. The examples that follow are but a few of the ways in which valuing activities can be incorporated into mental health education. Many of the other valuing strategies described in Chapter 3 can also be adapted to this content area.

Values Grid

This technique requires students to give priority to their values and publicly affirm them. The sixteen traits below should be placed in the grid, one trait per cell. When the values grid is completed, there will be four traits valued very highly, four highly, four mildly, and four for which there are no opinions. The following traits can be used:

1. peaceful
2. kind
3. open
4. tactful
5. confident
6. courteous
7. fearful
8. masculine
9. feminine
10. anxious
11. careful
12. materialistic
13. happy
14. lonely
15. popular
16. religious

A discussion of the completed grids should be concerned with the relationship between the placement of the traits and the students' own lives. The following questions are suggested for discussion:

1. Which of the traits that you valued "very highly" do you possess?
2. Which of these traits do you hope to possess in five years?
3. Of the "very highly" valued traits that you do not possess, how might you plan to acquire them? Who can help?
4. How many of the "very highly" valued traits does your best friend possess?
5. Why did you express "no opinion" about the four traits in that column?

Values Continuum

In this activity each student is asked to reflect on the following 10 statements and then identify where each statement would fit on the continuum line.

Agree	Neutral	Disagree

1. A friend should not criticize you.
2. Everyone should learn how to relax.
3. People should not keep secrets about themselves.
4. First impressions are usually accurate.
5. Feelings are private and should not be expressed.
6. It is difficult to receive a compliment graciously.
7. Doing things is more important than whom you're doing them with.

8. People need privacy.
9. Stress can be a positive influence.
10. When anxiety develops, tranquilizers should be taken.

Proud Statement

This is an activity which, if the students have developed trust and honest communication with one another, can help to identify values related to mental health, and which can be emotionally very touching. Students are asked to complete the statement, "I am proud that I . . ." and take turns telling the rest of the students how they responded. As stated previously, the students usually become more thoughtful and appreciative of their own worth and the value of their classmates as a result of this exercise.

Values Ranking

The process of ordering value statements by their importance, is an important component of the valuing process. The following groupings relate to mental health and can be used to identify and clarify values in that area:

1. popular	1. open	1. anxious
2. honest	2. secretive	2. calm
3. reliable	3. ashamed	3. excited
1. success	1. child	1. pets
2. happiness	2. adult	2. people
3. pride	3. senior citizen	3. things

Values Sheet

The values sheet consists of a provocative statement and a series of questions related to that statement with application to the students' personal lives. Here is a values sheet for mental health education:

Directions

Read the following statement and then answer the questions below honestly and thoughtfully.

Paul is a friend of Todd's. When Todd stopped dating Nancy because, as he said, "Nancy isn't good-looking enough," Paul called Todd aside.

"You are too concerned with what other people think," said Paul. "It was a mean thing to drop Nancy because other people might not find her attractive. She has a great personality and is real fun to be with."

"Mind your own business," said Todd. "If you were a good friend you'd understand how important it is for me to have the other guys and girls think well of me. How can they think I'm cool if I date an unattractive girl?"

Questions

1. Do you know anybody like Todd? Describe him or her.
2. Have you ever felt rejected like Nancy must have felt? When?
3. How could you make someone who feels rejected feel better?
4. What have you learned because of this exercise?

SUMMARY

The reader will note that this chapter does not concentrate on mental illness or what might be termed "Freudianism." Rather, the concern is for mental *health,* and the learning experiences described are consistent with that emphasis. In a preventive education program, such as health education, the focus should be one of prevention of illness through the maintenance of health. The rationale for the study of illness should be related to its prevention and not its treatment. Consequently, this chapter presents activities designed to prevent feelings of alienation and self-deprecation through the exploration of feelings toward oneself and others, which will better one's mental health status and decrease feelings of loneliness and isolation.

The learning experiences are directed at the development and maintenance of each student's mental health status, rather than an academic, generalized study of mental health. An outcome of such an approach is a much closer-knit group of classmates, better rapport between teacher and students, and a more efficient group of learners when subsequent health content areas are studied.

REFERENCES

1. Daniel I. Malamud and Solomon Machover, *Toward Self-Understanding: Group Techniques in Confrontation* (Springfield, Ill.: Charles C. Thomas, 1965), pp. 247–248.
2. This material is available from the Agency for Instructional Television; Box A, Bloomington, Indiana 47401.

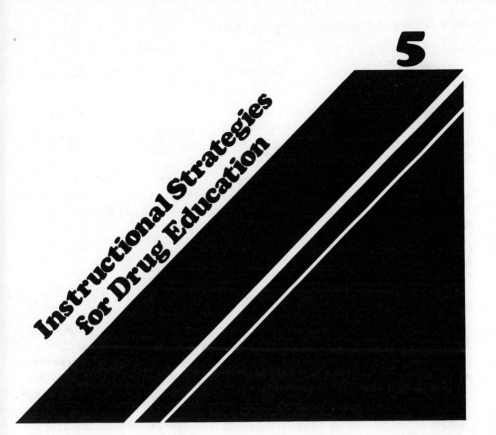

5

Instructional Strategies
for Drug Education

T he quest for a solution to the "drug problem" in our society has been unending. Unfortunately, simplistic solutions have been proposed for a very complex situation. As a result, no one is assured that any one method of drug education is more effective than any other. There are, however, a number of research reports and supported hypotheses of experts in drug education upon which to base a sound theory of drug education and a methodology consistent with that theory.

THE PIMPLE THEORY*

To better understand the kind of drug education which I will discuss, it will be helpful to employ an analogy which, though admittedly not physiologically sound, will crystallize some of the thoughts presented. Imagine a pimple roaming about a body seeking a place to surface. From head to toe the pimple roams until a potential place to appear is sighted. Now the person about whose body we are talking, deciding not to allow any pimples to surface, places his hand over the location the pimple seeks. The hand presses down hard and the pimple pushes up with all its might. Suddenly realizing there are only two hands to protect abundant potential "surfacing spots," the pimple gives up the fight and proceeds to an unprotected area at which it surfaces unmolested.

Health educators seem to be pressing down in isolated areas (drug abuse, health faddism, juvenile delinquency, and sexual misbehavior, for example) much as the hand attempts to prevent the pimple from surfacing. Unfortunately, even when the dam can be diked and drug abuse prevented, the water will pour through another opening. It is therefore recommended here that the underlying cause of drug abuse be determined and responded to, rather than the drug behavior itself. If one were able to eliminate the pimple (or the *causes* of drug abuse), then one wouldn't have to protect all parts of the body (or the sum total of potential unhealthy and/or antisocial *behaviors*) because there would be nothing left to surface.

What are these pimples which lead to such seemingly irrational behavior as drug abuse? Granted, there may be severe psychological problems associated with the use of particular addictive drugs. However, the causes of drug abuse to which I will refer have implications for a *preventive* drug program; i.e., drug education.

For several reasons, poverty can be disregarded as a cause of drug abuse. First, the economic background of students is a given element and nonmanipulative. Second, as will be discussed in the following pages, it is the *outcomes*

* This section is adapted from testimony presented by the author before the New York State Assembly Subcommittee on Drug Control, October 24, 1973.

of poverty rather than the condition itself that contribute to drug abuse. And third, the incidence of drug abuse among the children of wealthy and well-known people is evidence that drug abuse is not a result of lack of material possessions alone.[1]

Similarly, lack of knowledge of the consequences of drug abuse can be ruled out as a prevalent cause. Witness that "the incidence of narcotic addiction in physicians varies from 30 to 100 times that in the general population . . ."[2] In an investigation of the psychosocial correlates of alcohol use among college students it was found that there was no significant difference in grades between regular and occasional alcohol consumers.[3] It seems that intelligence or academic achievement is not related to abuse of drugs.

It has been suggested elsewhere that a negative concept of oneself *is* related to drug abuse. Levy, for instance, states:

> The users of the non-narcotic drugs seem to be doing more than just avoiding the pains and conflicts of living. They are seeking some way of overcoming their feelings of inadequacy and differentness. They have not been able to cope with existence satisfactorily. They feel unfulfilled and want meaningful experiences. They desperately want answers to the existential questions of: Who am I? What am I doing here? Where am I going? and How am I going there?[4]

Another researcher, after studying the smoking behavior of teenagers, concluded that "of all the variables examined in this study, these two peer smoking behavior variables best differentiate smokers from nonsmokers."[5] The two variables referred to were whether best friends or other pals smoked. The influence of peer behavior upon drug behavior evidently is an important one.

It has been found that a relationship exists between feelings of alienation (i.e., powerlessness, normlessness, and social isolation) and the use of marijuana and other drugs. After finding this relationship in an investigation of college students' use of marijuana, Harris states:

> Most important in applying the results of this study is reduction of the alienation which contributes to marijuana usage. The health educator, counselor, administrator, parent, or any other individual dealing with today's young people plays a role with the positive or negative effect on the student who feels isolated, powerless, and where guides for behavior in the form of specific values are lacking. For health educators, in particular, factual information alone is not sufficient to combat the increase in drug use on campus. Students need to feel that they are not alone, that decisions they make do influence the future, and values do exist which can influence decisions about drug usage.[6]

As causes of drug abuse that schools can respond to, we have considered: poor self-concept, negative peer influence, alienation, and values confusion. It is these causes, these underlying motivations and correlates of drug misbehavior, to which drug education programs should respond. To do so would not necessarily require discussion of physiological consequences of drug abuse, though such a discussion might be helpful. What would be required is a group leader, a teacher with knowledge of group dynamics and a command of learning experiences which will decrease feelings of alienation, clarify values, and increase students' concepts of self. These prerequisites are, it is sad to say, not always competencies of graduates of teacher training institutions. What is required, therefore, is a retraining of drug educators, and teachers in general, to make them more responsive to the *human* and less responsive to the *content* they are teaching.

It seems appropriate to conclude this section with a letter sent on the opening day of school to teachers from their principal:

Dear Teacher,

I am a survivor of a concentration camp. My eyes saw what no man should witness:

Gas chambers built by learned engineers. Children poisoned by educated physicians. Infants killed by trained nurses. Women and babies shot and burned by high school and college graduates.

So, I am suspicious of education.

My request is: Help your students become human. Your efforts must never produce learned monsters, skilled psychopaths, educated Eichmanns. Reading, writing, arithmetic are important, only if they serve to make our children more humane.[7]

The exercises to follow are designed to respond to the person rather than the drug.

PEER GROUP EXERCISES

One of the most pervasive factors related to drug misbehavior is peer group influence. The following exercises are designed to explore the existence of peer group pressure, how influential it is, how to react to negative peer pressure, and how to employ this phenomenon for beneficial purposes.

Reversed Seats

The effect of peer pressure is so impressive that students often engage in ridiculous behaviors because of this influence. To demonstrate this point, the teacher should send five student volunteers out of the classroom on a pretense of picking up pamphlets for distribution to the class. The faculty member to whom these students are sent should know they are coming and should delay them for several minutes. In the meantime, the teacher tells the class that: (1) when those students return, the class will continue its discussion as usual; (2) some time later, upon a signal from the teacher (perhaps pulling on the ear), the class members will sit on their desks and face the rear of the room; and (3) the conversation will continue just as if nothing had happened. Invariably several of the volunteers who weren't "clued in" will leave their seats and sit on their desks facing the rear. Often at least one volunteer will refuse to perform what he or she believes to be such a ridiculous act.

The students who left the room in search of pamphlets should then explain to the class:

a. How they felt when everyone sat on their desks facing the rear.

b. What they thought about before deciding whether to do what the class was doing or not go along with the class.

c. What they think they should have done when the class sat on their desks.

The students should discuss generalizations which can be drawn from this exercise and how peer group pressure influences behavior all the time. They should cite specific instances when their behavior was influenced by peers in spite of their own desires. The beneficial aspects of peer group pressure should not be overlooked in such a discussion. For instance, laws might be viewed as peer influence, but necessary and beneficial.

Paper-Bagging

The desire to impress our peers is so strong that we often are embarrassed to admit to a lack of experience. To explore this statement further, ask the class several questions during a large group discussion. These questions should be of a somewhat embarrassing, threatening, or revealing nature. For example:

a. How many use drugs?

b. How many have seen a person of the opposite sex naked?

c. How many have a problem with pimples?

d. How many have parents who argue a lot?

For each of these questions, record the number of students who raise their hands. Next, ask the students to place paper bags (provided by the students or the instructor) over their heads so that no one can see anyone else in the class. Then ask the same questions again, and again record the responses to each question. The count after the bags are on the heads is usually different from the earlier count, when everyone could see how everyone else responded. When the counts have been made, the students should discuss how they felt when the questions were read, both before and after the paper bags were in place. As with other exercises in this book, generalizations for daily behavior should be elicited.

Commercial Collaging

Some of the most energetic and carefully organized efforts to affect behavior by using the desire to impress one's peers are made by the advertising and marketing complexes. The nature of their efforts has been documented elsewhere.[8] To further analyze the extent and use of peer group influence, students can be asked to examine advertisements appearing in local newspapers and magazines. Those advertisements utilizing peer group influence can be cut out and used to create a collage for display in the classroom or elsewhere in the school building. Students may also find interest in creating their own posters counteracting the message of the advertisements. For example, an ad implying that the smoking of cigarettes will help one to become a he-man or beauty contest winner, might be placed beside a student-created collage of pictures of unattractive people smoking cigarettes in unappealing settings.

Commercial Recording

Since advertisements are not exclusive to the written medium, television and radio appeals to status in peer groups should also be investigated. One way to accomplish this is to have students agree to listen to a radio or television station for three hours on a Saturday morning, and record, in writing or on tape, instances of peer group pressure. Such recordings should be discussed in class the following Monday. To acquire a more complete picture, it is recommended that different students be assigned to listen to different television channels and radio stations. In this manner it will be possible to generalize to television and radio as a whole, and not be limited to data from only a few stations.

An analysis of the data brought to class by students will indicate that all ages are subject to peer group influence. The students might want to develop a school play, display case, or poster describing what they have learned from this activity.

Commercial Creating

While examination and analysis are useful learning activities, a more complicated behavior is creation. Using the knowledge and insight gleaned from Commercial Collaging and Commercial Recording, the class can be asked to create commercials themselves. These commercials must:

a. Use peer group influence appeals.
b. Advocate the nonabuse of drugs.
c. Be appropriate for the students' age group.
d. Be suitable for presentation over the school's public address system.

Subsequently, a drug education week can be established in the school and five commercials, chosen by a total class decision, can be broadcast over the school's public address system each morning (one each day).

Staged Argument

Rather like Reversed Seats, this activity demonstrates the effect of peer group pressure on decision-making. The teacher selects four students who enjoy the class and thinks up some pretext for them to leave the room. While they are gone, the teacher instructs the class to stage an argument with him or her about how bad the course is. When those who left the room return, the other students are also to attempt to solicit their active support in the argument. Usually those who left the room will either verbally support their classmates or remain silent. In any case, they will seldom support the teacher regardless of their beliefs.

A subsequent discussion of this activity will reveal the feelings of differentness, bewilderment, and loneliness experienced by those not in on the secret. The desire to alleviate these feelings is often the motivation for not expressing support for the teacher. If some do support the teacher, an examination of their motivations will prove interesting and informative.

Classroom Visitations

Though this exercise is often logistically difficult, a teacher who can arrange to have students observe others in the school or another school for some length of time, will be doing a service for those in his or her charge. Perhaps students can observe a class in a gymnasium, jot down notes from observations in the school cafeteria, watch others in the school library, or sit in on another class. In any of these situations, observers will frequently see behavior motivated by a need for peer approval. Probably the best environment to observe is a primary grade classroom where children are less sophisticated in hiding the reasons for their actions. After observations have been made and instances of behavior resulting from a need for peer approval recorded, the class should discuss the results of this activity.

Videotaping Plays

The use of videotape equipment and film-making equipment offers endless possibilities for contributing to the health instructional process. In one such endeavor, students might videotape playlets that demonstrate how need for peer approval may influence students to use drugs. These tapes might then be played for younger children as part of their drug education offerings. Students who create these videotapes should visit with the younger children as the tapes are shown to answer questions about the message being conveyed.

It would also prove valuable to videotape plays describing the results of several of the Peer Group Exercises described in this chapter. Such tapes could even be employed with teachers in an in-service educational activity. Thus, students would be teaching their teachers. Similarly, if these tapes were shown to parents during an evening set aside for such an occasion, students would, in effect, be educating their parents. What a revolutionary concept: teachers being taught by their students, and parents being educated by their children.

CROSSWORD PUZZLE

Although the cognitive aspects of drug education have been overemphasized in some health education programs, knowledge about drugs might best be considered a necessary but not sufficient condition to affect drug behavior. The task of the health instructor is to explore such knowledge with his or her students in an educationally sound setting with little threat of negatively affecting the variables cited at the beginning of this chapter. One excellent means for cognitive learning is the crossword puzzle. The reader may want to develop puzzles more apropos to his or her local situation than the example provided in Fig. 5.1.

DEBATES

One of the most valuable techniques for actively involving students in the learning process is the debate. A word of caution is in order, however. Often debates result in a discourse of ignorance due to insufficient planning on the part of the teacher and/or a lack of commitment on the part of the student debaters. A debate is not a loosely conducted experience but rather a highly structured activity. Several formats for debating have been proposed, but regardless of which format is chosen, consideration should be given to:

1. length of time for initial presentation,
2. length of time for rebuttal,
3. sequence for presentations and rebuttals,
4. length of time for closing statements,
5. procedures, if any, for audience participation, and
6. means and criteria for selecting a winner if one is to be chosen.

The time allowed for initial presentations, rebuttals, and closing statements will depend on the number of debaters and the length of the class. Assuming four debaters (two pro and two con) and a 40-minute class period, the following time allocations and sequence are recommended:

1. Initial presentation—four minutes per speaker (total: sixteen minutes).
2. Rebuttal after all initial presentations have been made—two minutes per speaker (total: eight minutes).
3. Questions from audience—eight minutes.
4. Closing statements—one minute for each debater (total: four minutes).
5. Class vote to determine winning team—one minute.
6. Miscellaneous—three minutes.

It can't be emphasized enough that debaters need ample time to research the topic and prepare a debating strategy. The teacher's role as facilitator neces-

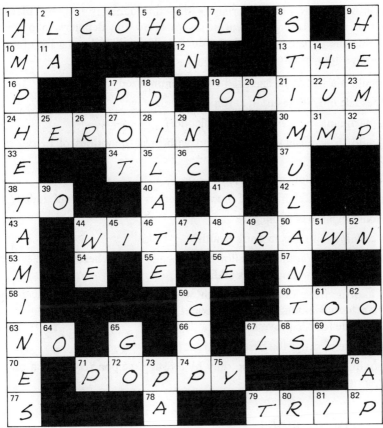

The crossword grid contains the following answers:

1. ALCOHOL 8. S 9. H
10. MA 12. N 13. THE
16. P 17. PD 19. OPIUM
24. HEROIN 30. MMP
33. E 34. TLC 37. U
38. TO 40. A 41. O 42. L
43. A 44. WITHDRAWN
53. M 54. E 55. E 56. E 57. N
58. I 59. C 60. TOO
63. NO 65. G 66. O 67. LSD
70. E 71. POPPY 76. A
77. S 78. A 79. TRIP

ACROSS

1. _____ mixed with barbiturates can cause death
10. Nickname for mother
13. Definite article
17. Abbr. for Police Department
19. A drug made from poppies
24. Abusers of this drug often get hepatitis
30. Abbr. for Marine Military Patrol
34. Abbr. for tender loving care
38. Toward
44. Reaction to the stoppage of an addictive drug
60. Also
63. Negative
67. Name for drug from a fungus on rye
71. Opium is made from the _____ plant
79. A drug-induced departure from reality

DOWN

1. A drug given for weight loss
2. Abbr. for Los Angeles
6. Covering
8. Classification of drugs which cause blood vessels to dilate
9. Common name for the marijuana plant found in India
14. To sing with your mouth closed
17. Slang for marijuana
18. To enlarge or get bigger
29. Abbr. for no charge
41. Poem of praise
44. Pl. of I
59. Abbr. for Constable on Patrol
61. Abbr. for Oh Dear!
65. Opposite of stop
73. Nickname for father
76. Abbr. for the Atlantic and Pacific Co.

Fig. 5.1 Drug Crossword Puzzle

sitates providing resource materials or directing debaters to them, planning for the debate well before the event so as to allow the debaters to prepare, and moderating the debate when it is conducted. The following is a list of drug education topics appropriate for debate:

1. Should marijuana be legalized (or decriminalized)?
2. Does use of LSD result in chromosomal damage?
3. Is marijuana more harmful than alcohol?
4. Should drug pushers apprehended with large quantities of heroin be jailed for life?
5. Do healthy people abuse drugs?
6. Is the housewife drug user more dangerous than the heroin addict?
7. Should cigarettes be illegal?
8. Is caffeine injurious to one's health?
9. Should heroin addicts be allowed to legally obtain heroin from government distributors to support their addiction?
10. If a drug were developed which would induce violent physical reactions when heroin enters the body, should this drug be placed in our water (as is fluoride for the prevention of tooth decay)?
11. Is the use of drugs the best way to get high?
12. Should aspirin be dispensed only by a druggist upon receipt of a physician's prescription?

BRAINSTORMING HIGHS

There are almost as many ways of getting "high" or "turning on" as there are people. An activity to demonstrate this concept utilizes the brainstorming approach. The brainstorming method is basically one in which students supply instant ideas that may be associated either closely or remotely with the problem being discussed. The basic rules for brainstorming are:

1. List ideas related to the problem as quickly as possible.
2. Do not criticize.
3. The more ideas, the better.
4. After all ideas are listed, combine and/or modify them.
5. From a discussion of the remaining ideas, decide on one or several solutions to the problem.

An example of the classroom use to which brainstorming might be applied will serve to further clarify this methodology. If, as part of a senior high school unit on mental health, the problem of what a male student should do upon being drafted to the Army is to be discussed, the brainstorming technique can be useful. As many ideas as possible can be solicited from the class (e.g., go into the Army, move to Canada, rob a gas station, appeal to the draft board, etc.) before a discussion of these ideas results in consensus on the appropriate re-action to a draft notice. Since criticism of ideas is barred until all ideas are listed, the insecure student is less threatened and therefore more verbally active when brainstorming is employed.

The many and varied means of getting "high" that were elicited through brainstorming could serve as a listing of alternatives to drug abuse. Some of the suggestions on this list will be judged inappropriate by the class when a discussion of the listing is undertaken. Some may be illegal, immoral, unethical, impractical, or impossible. But the remaining suggestions might present mean-ingful choices for youngsters who have heretofore been unable to identify ways, other than drugs, to get excited about life.

CLASSROOM VISITORS

Whether due to school budget restrictions, excessive distance to the site one wishes to visit, or of the inability of the site to handle the number of students in the class, field trips are not always possible. An alternative to visiting the site is to have someone from the site visit the class. Classroom visitors offer a dimen-sion to learning that teachers or fellow students often can not offer. With a frame of reference not possessed by students or teachers, visitors to the classroom tend to create interest by the dissimilarity to everyday classroom activity and their expertise relative to the purpose for their visit. It would be naive to assume that every visitor a class invites will provide a worthwhile use of class time. Some visitors may be knowledgeable but very poor speakers, some visitors may be excellent speakers but not very knowledgeable, and, lo and behold, some speak-ers may be neither knowledgeable nor well-spoken. It is therefore recommended that the teacher or a representative group of the students meet with the invited guest prior to the visitation so as to:

1. allow the class representative to assess the potential of the visit,
2. acquaint the speaker with the interest and knowledge level of the group about the speaker's topic,
3. obtain from the visitor ideas for preparing the class for his or her visitation, and
4. plan with the guest the format his or her visit will take (lecture, question-and-answer, round-table discussion, etc.).

Visitors for drug education classes could be chosen from among counselors from neighborhood counseling centers, personnel of detoxification units, representa-tives from several organizations which offer varying modes of treatment (group therapy, methadone withdrawal or maintenance, psychoanalysis, self-help communities, etc.), and police officers from narcotics squads.

CASE STUDY

Often learning that derives from the analysis of how others have behaved can be meaningful. Role-playing has been cited as one experience in which the analysis of the actions and reactions of others can enhance empathy and understanding. Analyses of case studies also enhances learning. The cases, or stories, can be read aloud by the teacher, shown on film, or written out for the students to read. Whatever the method, a story is presented and analyzed, and conclusions are drawn. By way of example, the teacher might read to the class a story of a teenager whose girlfriend has deserted him, whose parents aren't responsive to his needs, to whom school is a "bummer," and who subsequently uses drugs to relieve himself of his frustrations. Students might then be asked how friends, parents, and teachers could have prevented the drug abuse; what other avenues of escape from one's frustrations there are; and what the implications of this story are for each of the students in the class. For the case study method to be accepted, the case must be relevant to the interests and/or needs of the students for whom it is intended. Stories from newspapers, books, related experiences, and vivid imaginations are several sources from which cases can be obtained. Regardless of the derivation of the case or cases to be employed, care should be taken to conclude the analysis of each case with a discussion of its implications to the participating students.

CRITICAL INCIDENT

Whereas the case study method of instruction utilizes a story with a beginning, middle, and end, the critical-incident approach does not supply an end to the story. The learner, therefore, is responsible for developing plausible endings for the story. This open-ended technique allows pupils to place themselves in a role that has been described and act out the end of that story as the student perceives it. The advantage of this methodology to the case study method is that students have to use their own creative abilities to end the story rather than react to a given ending. The nature of the case when employing critical incidents must be such that at the point at which the story ends a decision is necessary (thus becoming the critical incident in the story). Steps suggested for the use of the critical incident technique are:

1. Reading the incident.
2. Acquiring or agreeing on assumptions about additional facts that are needed.
3. Discussing the major issues.
4. Summarizing the issues.

5. Each individual recording his or her own reaction to the critical incident.

6. Forming groups to react to the critical incident.*

As can be readily determined, the critical incident technique can be used in conjunction with sociodrama as well as with other methodologies yet to be discussed.

Here are two examples of critical incidents which can be used with drug education classes:

> Janice was fourteen years old last June when she completed junior high school. Her best friend (really her *only* friend) had to move out of town with her parents at that point and, consequently, Janice had the loneliest, most miserable summer of her life. It was September when Janice entered a strange school (the high school) without anyone to whom she could confide her apprehensions. She sat next to Paula in English class and when Paula asked her to go with her to a party that weekend, Janice was ecstatic. When they entered the party, Janice noticed that there were a number of people smoking marijuana. Soon Paula took a marijuana cigarette from her pocketbook and asked Janice to smoke one too. Janice thought about her loneliness and then about the marijuana. Then Janice. . . .

> Philip was bored. He wasn't very good at sports, did poorly in his school work, and did not have any real good friends. Realizing that his life was unexciting and that the future didn't look much better, Philip decided to turn within himself for excitement. He knew where all the "dopers" hung out and went there to see if he could get a drug that would help him forget about his problems. When he reached the street corner where the crowd who used drugs usually spent their time, Philip saw Jeff. Since he used to be in Philip's class before he decided to drop out of school, and Philip knew he used drugs, Jeff was the perfect person for Philip to talk with. When Philip explained his situation, Jeff said, "I've got just the thing, baby. LSD will trip you right through yourself. You'll have a religious experience, man, with all sorts of colors and shapes. Real spaced out. What do you say? Want some?" Philip said. . . .

STRENGTH BOMBARDMENT

One of the suspected correlates to drug abuse is poor concept of self. It is hypothesized that students who do not have high regard for themselves and their opinions are more apt to be influenced by peers than those with a positive self-concept. Since the desire for peer status is also a suspected correlate to drug abuse, it seems reasonable to seek to improve students' self-concepts so that *they* can decide whether or not to use drugs with as little negative interference from their friends as possible. Strength Bombardment is one means to improve self-esteem.

---

* Adapted from Cyrus Mayshark and Roy Foster, *Methods in Health Education: A Workbook Using the Critical Incident Technique* (St. Louis: The C. V. Mosby Co., 1966), pp. 6–7. Used by permission.

If possible, organize the class so that the students are seated in a circle. It is important that the seating formation be circular rather than square or oblong, since only a circular seating arrangement allows each participant to see each other participant. One student becomes the focus of the group's attention, and the class' comments are directed only to that student. The other students are told to tell that student as many positive statements about him- or herself as they can develop in five minutes. The statements, however, must be true; false flattery is not the intention. Though it is easier to think of positive statements for some students than others, everyone has some good traits. Therefore, every student can, at one time or another, serve as the "focus."

The results of this exercise are severalfold. First, the bond between the "focus" and his or her classmates becomes stronger. They tend to feel better about each other than before the exercise. Second, students who have always felt useless, worthless, and inconsequential begin to think that they have something to contribute to the class and to others outside of the class. For perhaps the very first time, these students have *focused* on their positive traits and have had others do so as well. It is not unusual for some students to have positive aspects of themselves, which they never knew existed, brought to their attention for the first time during this activity. Lastly, an atmosphere of camaraderie, which is conducive to subsequent humanistic health education strategies, is created as a result of Strength Bombardment.

It is recommended that Strength Bombardment be employed for short periods of time (perhaps two students in any one session) over the history of the class. An observant teacher who can perceive when his or her students are "down in the dumps" can employ this exercise to save the day for them. Strength Bombardment is also an excellent means to end a class session which has concerned itself with a topic of controversy. When students argue a point on such topics, they often come away angry. Strength Bombardment can restore the desired class atmosphere and aid students who have argued to feel better about each other.

FORCED ARGUING

This exercise is related to *maintenance* of positive self-concept once it is developed. It provides students the opportunity to practice feeling good about themselves and their opinions, in spite of someone else's negative remarks or feelings. This activity is organized in small groups (from four to six students per group) and requires each student to think of something about which he or she feels good. On becoming "it," each student tells the group what he or she feels good about. The group's task is to take the opposite position from the student, and argue with him or her. Name-calling *is* allowed. "It's" task is to maintain his or her good feelings in spite of the negative remarks of the other group members.

A variation of this activity is to have those who are "it" relate to the group negative feelings they have about themselves, some things they've done, defeats they have experienced, or personal weaknesses they perceive about themselves. The group's task is then to argue against "it's" self-depreciation. In this manner, each student in the group will feel better about himself or herself in spite of some negative characteristic or experience which has previously led to some self-depreciation.

THERMOMETER

A means of soliciting opinions and positions from students in a more exotic fashion than just by asking for them is to take the class' temperature on certain issues. This procedure calls for the teacher, or a student, to draw a long thermometer on a sheet of paper which will be spread out on the classroom floor. If the custodian allows it, chalk can be used to draw the thermometer on the floor. Even paint can be employed if this exercise is going to be used often.

Next the teacher raises an issue (e.g., arrest of alcoholics) and asks the class "how hot" they get over this issue. The "hotter" or more bothered they are about an issue, the higher they stand on the thermometer. The less concerned they feel about the issue, the cooler they are toward it, and therefore, the lower they stand on the thermometer.

A variation of this exercise is to distribute paper to the students upon which appears a picture of a thermometer and a statement of the issue printed across the top. In this case, students are asked to place an × at the appropriate spot on the thermometer, indicating how concerned they are about the issue. In small groups they discuss why they placed the × where they did.

Some issues which can be used for drug education are:

1. People smoking in a room where nonsmokers are present.
2. Pregnant women smoking cigarettes.
3. Methadone maintenance.
4. Involuntary use of antabuse.
5. Aversive therapy (e.g., electric shock administered when an alcoholic reaches for a drink).
6. Legalization of marijuana.

INTERVIEWS

Students often come in contact with problem drinkers, users of illegal drugs, and cigarette smokers. Such is the state of affairs in our country. Rather than deny this fact, a good health educator will use it for the betterment of his or her students. After studying drugs and related issues, it would be worthwhile for students to interview users of drugs (alcohol, illegal drugs, misused legal drugs, tobacco, properly used legal drugs) to determine:

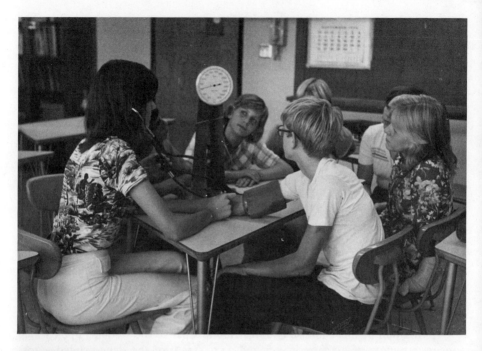

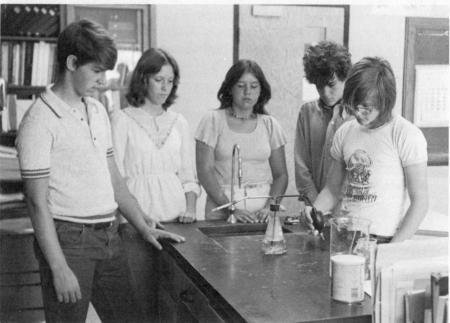

Laboratory experiments are good ways of developing interest in health content.

1. Their motivations for abusing the drug.
2. Whether they abuse other drugs and how.
3. When they first started abusing drugs and which drug that was.
4. Whether their lives have changed as a result of abusing drugs.
5. Whatever else is on the minds of the students in the class.

Other interviews might be with other students in the school or community, parents, physicians, psychologists, school nurses, or public health officials. It should be remembered that the object of this activity is for students to see how what they have learned in an enclosed environment (the school) applies to the community at large.

LABORATORY EXPERIMENTATION

How many times as youngsters did we hear the challenge, "Prove it"? One technique teachers can use to "prove it" is laboratory experimentation. Rather than lecture on the effects of nicotine in the body, for instance, teachers can extract nicotine from a pack of cigarettes, inject it into a mouse, and have the class observe the mouse's sluggish, uncoordinated movements and eventual convulsions. A subsequent dissection of the mouse will show the stimulating effect of nicotine upon the heart, since the heart will beat longer in a dead mouse injected with nicotine than will the heart of a dead mouse into which nicotine has not been injected.

It may be possible for the health educator to coordinate his or her activities with those of the science teacher during laboratory experimentation sessions. Facilities and equipment, if shared, can be provided at a lower cost to the school (and therefore more easily justified as an expenditure) than if the science and health education teachers did not correlate their activities.

VALUING ACTIVITIES

Drug education provides many opportunities for the teacher to use valuing exercises. Some examples of how the consideration of the relationship between values and drug behavior can be conducted are presented in this section. The teacher is encouraged, however, to adapt still other values clarification activities to drug education.

Values Ranking

Asking students to rank their preferences related to drug behavior will help them to identify and clarify values of which they may not have been previously aware. Some groupings that can be used for rank ordering are shown on the next page.

1. drug pusher	1. to think well of oneself
2. drug addict	2. to be thought well of by friends
3. drug grower	3. to be thought well of by adults

1. physical health	1. high	1. drink beer
2. social health	2. straight	2. smoke marijuana
3. mental health	3. cool	3. pop pills

Values Statements

Another means of studying values as they relate to drug behavior is to have students complete sentences which indicate values and then discuss their responses. Examples of such sentences are:

1. I use drugs when_____
2. My body_____
3. My friends_____
4. Marijuana _____
5. To be high is_____
6. To be straight is_____
7. To be cool means_____
8. Pills_____
9. My head_____
10. I feel alienated when_____

Values Judgment

Case studies can be combined with valuing to produce an activity that will elicit value judgments. In the following example, several values are manifested in the behavior of the story's characters. After reading the story, the students are asked to list the characters in the order in which they like them.

> John was a drug pusher, but not the ordinary kind. When Mary came to John for some drugs, John gave them to her even though Mary had no money to pay for them. He gave her a nickel bag of marijuana ($5.00 worth) and some cocaine to snort. The next day Mary felt it was unfair to hit John up for some more free drugs, so she broke into Frank's grocery store and stole $75.00 from the cash register. However, a policeman saw Mary leave and chased after her. When he caught her and asked Frank if he would press charges, Frank hesitated. He whispered to Mary that he would drop the charges if Mary slept with him that night. Mary was angered to hear Frank's request and slapped his face. When the policeman saw this, he charged Mary with assault as well as robbery.
>
> Place the names of John, Mary, Frank and the policeman in the order in which you like them. First listed will be the one you most like, second listed will be

the one you like next best, and so on until the last one listed is the one you
like the least.

Values Continuum

Having students place themselves somewhere between two extremes of an issue
and discussing the reasons for placing themselves where they did, is still another
means of investigating values. This technique is called the values continuum. Two
values continua which may be used in drug education are:

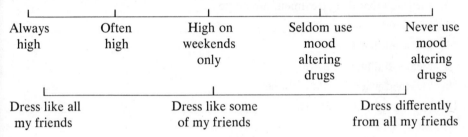

Always high	Often high	High on weekends only	Seldom use mood altering drugs	Never use mood altering drugs

Dress like all my friends	Dress like some of my friends	Dress differently from all my friends

The first example presented relates specifically to drug behavior and, when
discussed, may indicate inconsistency or confusion in values. For instance, if
some students have previously indicated a value for independence quite typical
of adolescence, their dependence on drugs may be cited as contrary to this professed value. The second example cited above relates to the influence of students'
peers upon their behavior. As has been stated earlier in this chapter, there exists
a relationship between students' behavior and that of their peers. The extent to
which this influence affects each student can be demonstrated with this values
continuum. The values inherent in this influence can then be examined.

Medicine Cabinet Inspection

Many times we have values which contradict one another and we must decide for
one at the expense of the other. An exercise to demonstrate this point requires
students to list everything they find in their medicine cabinets at home. Once
these lists are developed, ask the following questions:

1. Did you find prescription drugs that were no longer needed? Does your family value money over safety?
2. Did you find many over-the-counter drugs for headaches? Does your family
   value quick relief over self-discipline?
3. Did you find mood altering drugs? Does your family value highs from sub-
   stances over highs from people and activity?
4. Were drugs out of the reach of children? Does your family value safety over
   convenience?

Learning Statements

At the conclusion of valuing activities, students can be asked to write paragraphs that begin with any of the following phrases:

1. I learned that drugs_____
2. I learned that people_____
3. I learned that isolation_____
4. I learned that getting high_____
5. I learned that drug treatment modalities_____
6. I learned that my values_____
7. I learned that I need_____
8. I learned that my health_____
9. I learned when people are lonely_____
10. I learned that friends often_____

CONCLUSION

In conclusion it should be noted that most of the learning experiences described in this chapter relate to objectives other than learning about drugs. Consistent with the opening statement of this chapter, drug abuse is not the problem, but only the symptom. The causes of the symptom are many and varied. Negative peer influence and values confusion were two of the causes of drug abuse to which the activities in this chapter were directed. Activities designed to affect poor self-concept and alienation, two other causes of drug abuse, were described in Chapter 4. In addition, learning experiences in which cognition about drugs could be achieved were also presented. Since many drug education programs ignore the psychosocial aspects of the "drug problem," however, the focus of this chapter has been to help the health educator better respond to those needs.

REFERENCES

1. United Press International, "Drugs and Children of Famous People," *Boston Globe,* August 6, 1970.
2. Associated Press, "AMA Units Ask Action Against 'Sick' Doctors," *Buffalo Evening News,* November 27, 1972, p. 6.
3. John Robinson and James Brown, *Psycho-Social Correlates of Alcohol Use Among University Students,* unpublished paper presented before the American School Health Association, October 14, 1973, Table 4.
4. Norman Levy, "The Use of Drugs by Teenagers for Sanctuary and Illusion," *New York State Narcotic Addiction Control Commission Reprints* **3** (no date), p. 4.

5. Richard Lannes, Franklin Banks, and Martin Keller. "Smoking Behavior in a Teenage Population: A Multivariate Conceptual Approach," *American Journal of Public Health* **62** (1972), p. 808.

6. Eileen M. Harris, "A Measurement of Alienation in College Student Marijuana Users and Non-users," *The Journal of School Health* **41,** 3 (1971), p. 133. Used by permission.

7. Source unknown.

8. Vance Packard, *The Hidden Persuaders* (New York: Simon & Schuster, 1957).

6

Instructional Strategies for Sex and Family Living Education

A

ided by the notoriety of Masters and Johnson's research (1966) and references to a sexual revolution, human sexuality has become a topic recently much discussed and researched. In fact, sexuality has achieved the status where one's sexual problems can be freely discussed with strangers via a telephone hot-line.[1] The need to develop such responses to sexual problems as hot-lines seems to indicate a discomfort with sexuality or misconceptions pertaining to sex. Welbourne states that:

> [there are] a lot of people who feel guilty or very anxious about sex because they are misinformed. They're living with a lot of delusions or myths. And their feeling can often be alleviated just by providing them with information about sex.[2]

An inspection of sources of sex information indicates that primary sources do not appear to be reliable. Thornburg, in two studies of sources of sex information, found that a majority of such information possessed by college women was obtained from peers and literature, whereas only 15 percent was acquired from schools and 21 percent from parents.[3] Thornburg's findings are consistent with those of other researchers.[4]

One response to the person who is misinformed and ill-at-ease about sex and sexuality has been the development of school sex education programs. Though some school districts are experiencing problems with these programs,[5] surveys indicate that parents agree that their childrens' schools should have a sex education program (83.8%) and that, generally speaking, sex education should be offered in the schools (88.4%). Only a small percentage of parents thought that: the teaching of sex education in schools will destroy the morals of children (4.6%), sex education should be given only in the home (4.3%), sex education in the schools is an invasion of family rights and privacy (6.4%), and most parents are capable of teaching their children about sex education (16.6%).[6]

A study of school administrators' attitudes toward sex education conducted in Texas is indicative of administrators' attitudes elsewhere in the United States. A majority of Texas school district superintendents agreed that the public school should assume the responsibility for educating their students about sexuality.[7]

The attitudes of these superintendents' seem to make sense when it is realized that students indicating "the school as their major source of (sex) information demonstrated a significantly higher degree of knowledge about sexuality than those students who listed parents or friends as the major source of information."[8]

In view of the easily documented need for sex and family life education, this chapter presents learning activities to aid health educators respond to the needs and interests of their students relative to sexuality. The chapter is divided into sections pertaining to *selected* aspects of sex and family life education, and should not be considered all-inclusive of content in this area. However, activities designed to raise issues of current societal concern are provided, as well as issues of longstanding study.

"NEED FOR" ACTIVITIES

The first three activities can be used to underline the need for sex and family life education. It will be assumed that the interest in such study has already been engendered (an assumption this writer feels confident in making).

Sexy Collage

One need only glance at newspaper and magazine advertisements to notice their appeals to sexual needs and desires. The "manly" man with the "sexy" woman enjoying a walk through the woods with a cigarette; the best thing (cigar) from Sweden since the blond; the bikinied girl standing beside a car; and the candy mint that is a breath freshener and results in the user kissing an attractive mate.

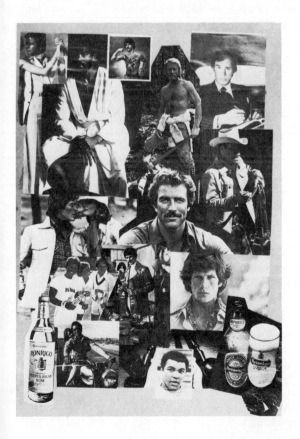

This is a picture of a Sexy Collage created by a student. The theme of this collage is "A Man Is." Note the ruggedness of the men depicted. This collage prompted a great deal of discussion.

Add to these the announcements of movies about student nurses who shouldn't but do, the husband and wife who should but don't, and the rest who wish they could but can't, and the result is a society whose sexual needs are continually exploited and conditioned.

When students are asked to create collages on large sheets of oak tag which reflect appeals to sex that appear in newspapers and magazines, they soon realize how such appeals influence their own behavior. The posting of these collages, and the opportunity for the class to view them, should be followed by small group discussions of how each student has been so influenced. Some topics to be used in these discussions are:

1. By which advertisement appealing to sexual needs were you recently influenced?
2. What did this advertisement make you do?
3. How was this advertisement presented to you? Television? Newspaper? Magazine? Would you have reacted differently if it were presented in one of the other two media?
4. What would you tell younger brothers or sisters to help them *not* be influenced by this advertisement the way you were?

Sex As . . .

Another manner in which the need for sex education can be demonstrated is to identify ways in which sex has been employed by the students, or how they feel it should be employed. The questionnaire below is designed for this purpose. It should be noted, however, that "sex" is not used synonymously with sexual intercourse or any other particular sexual behavior. "Sex" might refer to flirting, wearing provocative clothing, or using a perfume designed for "ambush." After the questionnaire is completed by each student, form small groups for a discussion of the manner in which sex is used as _____.

SEX AS[9]

Directions: Try and identify with this list of "Sex As" and pick those phrases which most represent your feelings. Try to identify with at least three. Place a + after the ones you choose.

___ Sex as purely playful activity
___ Sex as a way to have babies
___ Sex as fun
___ Sex an expression of hostility
___ Sex as punishment
___ Sex as a mechanical duty
___ Sex as an outlet from physiological or psychological tension
___ Sex as a protection against alienation

___ Sex as a way of overcoming separateness or loneliness
___ Sex as a way to communicate deep involvement in the welfare of another
___ Sex as a form of "togetherness"
___ Sex as a reward
___ Sex as a revenge
___ Sex as an act of rebellion
___ Sex as an experiment
___ Sex as an adventure
___ Sex as a deceit
___ Sex as a form of self-enhancement
___ Sex as an exploitation for personal gain
___ Sex as proof

Go back over the list and place an × after those you have used but are not happy with.

Hot Line

It is now time for the reader to apply some self-appraisal. This next activity requires an instructor more comfortable with sex and sexuality than is usual for a health educator. It also requires a teacher with a great deal of knowledge about sex-related topics. This activity, Hot Line, begins when the teacher announces to the health education classes that a certain telephone has been designated for their calls between certain hours of the day. The telephone number and times for calls (perhaps during the teacher's preparation period or right after the students are dismissed for the day) should be written on the blackboard and each student *required* to write these in his or her notebook. Some students might feel embarrassed to write down the numbers unless *all* are required to do so. The instructor then explains that any questions they want to ask which relate to sex or family life, no matter how silly, will be answered by the teacher on the telephone at the prescribed times. The teacher should emphasize that the identities of the callers will remain unknown.

As can be expected, such an activity will allow Johnny Joker to call and ask an embarrassing or insulting question. However, if the teacher can live through such calls, other callers will display a naiveté and lack of sophistication and knowledge that will evidence the need for sex and family life education. At the same time, students too embarrassed to ask questions in class will be provided the opportunity to ask these questions anonymously.

Question Box

The Question Box has a purpose similiar to that of the Hot Line—namely, to provide an anonymous means for students to ask, and have answered, questions related to sex and family life. Such a box should be placed in a convenient location so as to allow students to place inside the box pieces of paper on which are written questions. The teacher should periodically, perhaps once a week, remove the questions from the box and provide class time for answering them. The following is a sample of the questions obtained by the Question Box technique in one junior high school:[10]

How do you know if you are a homosexual?

What is the most common thing that goes wrong with childbirth?

Why don't some boys between the ages of ten and fourteen notice girls because they are so interested in sports (sic)?

Does a boy have anything happen to him? Not a menstruation period but maybe something like that?

Why doesn't a man know that he is a father after being in bed and (sic) given it to her (the baby). But instead when she goes to the doctor she finds out, then comes back and tells the father and it is a complete shock to him.

What's a Kotex?

If you have a discharge, does that necessarily mean you have V.D.?

If a woman is pregnant and she is on drugs, and she is still taking drugs during the pregnancy will this affect the baby?

Is there something wrong? Mine (menstrual period) comes every 21 days.

What is rape?

Can a woman have a child after a miscarriage?

MASCULINE/FEMININE ROLES

One of the topics currently being debated is the role of women and, consequently, the role of men in our society. To simplify the debate, behaviorists believe that much of sexual role determination is learned behavior. An example: boys learn to be aggressive and girls learn to be passive because of the games they play. The "naturists" believe that the sexual role is inherited, or related to hormonal secretions. That is, males are more aggressive than females because they have a greater amount of androgen. The following activities will help the teacher involve the students in the study of sexual and/or gender roles.

Sex Riddle

To highlight the prevalence of sterotypic thinking relative to sex roles, the teacher should distribute the following handout:*

---

* Excerpted from *Go To Health,* by Communications Research Machines, Inc. Copyright © 1973 by Communications Research Machines, Inc. Reprinted by permission of Delacorte Press.

A father and his son were involved in a car accident in which the father was killed and the son was seriously injured. The father was pronounced dead at the scene of the accident and his body taken to a local mortuary. The son was taken by ambulance to a local hospital and was immediately wheeled into an operating room. A surgeon was called. Upon seeing the patient, the attending surgeon exclaimed, "Oh, my God, it's my son!" Can you explain this? (Keep in mind the father who was killed in the accident is not a stepfather, nor is the attending physician the boy's stepfather.) Think about the "riddle" for a few minutes. If you think you have the answer, write it on a sheet of paper.

The answer is then read: The surgeon was the boy's mother.

The inability of most (if not all) of the class to conceive of the surgeon as a woman can then be discussed. Such questions as the following should be posed:

1. What other jobs are usually thought of as masculine? Feminine?
2. Can women (men) perform these jobs well?
3. Why do you think these jobs have been assigned to women (men)?
4. What is your thinking regarding sex-role stereotyping?

Imaginary Mirror

With the purpose of further exploring stereotypes associated with sex role, students can be asked to give their conceptions of masculine and feminine in a unique manner. The teacher asks the students to close their eyes and imagine that they are looking in a magic mirror. In that mirror they see someone of the opposite sex (do not mention the age of the image they see). The class is told that they can see everything about that person: what he or she looks like, how he or she functions socially, the I.Q. of the image, and the emotional responses the image exhibits. The class is then given 20 minutes to describe, in writing, the image they saw relative to the following four categories:

1. physically
2. emotionally
3. intellectually
4. socially

After the descriptions have been written, volunteers should be allowed to read their descriptions to the total group of students. When six descriptions have been read for each sex, the teacher then asks the class to pick out the points they have in common. It will be noted that the females imagined by the male students were young, beautiful, sweet, cute, bright, cried easily, etc., whereas the female students will have imagined their male image to be brave, strong, handsome, athletic, shy, a show-off, etc. A discussion of sexual stereotyping will then be meaningful and relate to the students' own stereotypes as opposed to discussing, with academic disguise, stereotypes in general.

Role Paradox

The male's concept of femininity and the female's concept of masculinity each have an effect on what the opposite sex becomes. An excellent means of analyzing this effect is to distribute a handout containing the quotation below. Allow time in class for the students to read the handout and jot down notes as they read. When everyone is done, form small groups to discuss the handout.[11]

> He is playing masculine. She is playing feminine. She is playing feminine *because* he is playing masculine. He is playing masculine *because* she is playing feminine.
>
> He is playing the kind of man that he thinks the kind of woman she is playing ought to admire. She is playing the kind of woman that she thinks the kind of man he is playing ought to desire.
>
> If he were not playing masculine, he might well be more feminine than she is— except when she is playing very feminine. If she were not playing feminine, she might well be more masculine than he—except when he is playing very masculine.
>
> So he plays harder. And she plays—softer.
>
> He wants to make sure that she could never be more masculine than he. She wants to make sure that he could never be more feminine than she. He therefore seeks to destroy the femininity in himself. She therefore seeks to destroy the masculinity in herself.
>
> She is supposed to admire him for the masculinity in him that she fears in herself. He is supposed to desire her for the femininity in her that he despises in himself.
>
> He desires her for her femininity which is *his* femininity, but which he can never lay claim to. She admires him for his masculinity which is *her* masculinity, but which she can never lay claim to. Since he may only love his own femininity in her, he envies her her femininity.
>
> Since she may only love her own masculinity in him, she envies him his masculinity.
>
> The envy poisons their love.
>
> He, coveting her unattainable femininity, decides to punish her. She, coveting his unattainable masculinity, decides to punish him. He denigrates her femininity —which he is supposed to desire and which he really envies—and becomes more aggressively masculine. She feigns disgust at his masculinity—which she is supposed to admire and which she really envies—and becomes more fastidiously feminine. He is becoming less and less what he wants to be. She is becoming less and less what she wants to be. But now he is more manly than ever, and she is more womanly than ever.
>
> Her femininity, growing more dependently supine, becomes contemptible. His masculinity, growing more oppressively domineering, becomes intolerable. At last she loathes what she has helped his masculinity to become. At last he loathes what he has helped her femininity to become.
>
> So far, it has all been very symmetrical. But we have left one thing out.

The world belongs to what his masculinity has become.

The reward for what his masculinity has become is power. The reward for what her feminity has become is only security which his power can bestow upon her.

If he were to yield to what her femininity has become, he would be yielding to contemptible incompetence. If she were to acquire what his masculinity has become, she would participate in intolerable coerciveness.

She is stifling under the triviality of her femininity. The world is groaning beneath the terrors of his masculinity.

He is playing masculine. She is playing feminine.

How do we call off the game?

Sex Role Dislikes/Likes

To begin a discussion of what boys dislike about girls and what girls dislike about boys, divide the class into two groups—one all male and the other all female. Have each group brainstorm what they dislike about the opposite sex. After 20 minutes of such activity, one male and one female are selected to read the list their group developed. An argument should then be developed between the two groups to allow the presenting of stereotypes related to sex role which are often believed and felt, but not often stated publicly.

The next class meeting, or the end of this class session if time permits, should be devoted to a similar activity, except that the focus should be on what is *liked* about the opposite sex. Any ill feelings associated with the first phase of this activity should be eliminated as a result of phase 2.

House Building

Whether innate or acquired, there are differences between males and females relative to a large number of issues. One means of demonstrating such differences is to ask students to compose a list of those things they would look for in buying or building a house. Only the five to ten most important considerations should be listed. When the lists are completed, randomly pair males with females and have the partners exchange lists. From the two lists before them, each pair must then develop *one* list of five considerations they agree are important in buying or building a house. Compromise will be necessary, as will a realization regarding those factors females look for in a house and those that males believe are important. Obviously there is some relationship in house building and life style. This relationship should be noted for the class by the instructor.

Sex Tasking

This is another activity which will illuminate sex role expectations and develop an appreciation of the sexual pigeonhole in which people are placed. It requires that girls list those tasks associated with "femaleness" which they desire to give up and those tasks associated with "maleness" which they would like to adopt. Similarly, boys should develop lists of "male tasks" they desire to drop and "female tasks" they desire to adopt. The two sets of lists should be compared in small groups for similarities. It will soon become evident that there are some tasks neither group wants to be responsible for and some tasks each group wants to adopt. The proposal of a reasonable and *just* solution to this dilemma should be the responsibility of the small groups .

The participation in Sex Tasking usually results in the posing of some of the following questions:

1. Why do women wash dishes?
2. Why do men take out the garbage?
3. Why do boys pay for the date?
4. Why are girls picked up on a date?
5. Why do women prepare the meals?
6. Why don't girls ask boys out on a date?
7. Why do women take care of the children while men work?
8. Why aren't girls' athletic teams as important as boys' athletic teams?

Head Tapes

Often a teacher will want to have students express their biases in a nonthreatening atmosphere. Head Taping allows students to attribute their biases and stereotypes to the role they're playing. The teacher divides the class into small groups of six members each. Strips of adhesive tape, upon which roles are written, are placed on the foreheads of each student without the student learning what role he or she is to play. Students can see the roles assigned to other students (since the roles are written on the tapes stuck to their foreheads) but cannot see their own role (since they cannot see their own foreheads). The group then engages in a conversation about society, and each group member is to treat the other group members as though they were the type of person identified on their head tapes. By way of example, if Johnny is to play a he-man, the word "he-man" would appear on the tape on his forehead. During the group conversation, the group is to react to whatever Johnny says or does as though he really were a he-man. The roles assigned should be as follows:

1. Sexy Susie
2. Athletic Abe
3. Intellectual Izzy
4. Masculine Madeline
5. Sissy Stanley
6. Ugly Augustine

As the conversation goes on, the participants are to write down their own roles when they think they know them. When all group members have guessed the role they have been assigned, the tapes are removed and the students determine whether or not their guesses were accurate. A discussion in small groups regarding why Sexy Susie, for example, was greeted with smiles while Ugly Augustine with disdain, will do much to help stereotypes surface. The teacher should conclude by stating that how one is treated often becomes a self-fulfilling prophecy. That is to say, if one is treated as though one is worthless, one will behave "worthlessly." If one is treated as a person of importance, one tends to behave "importantly." Similarly, if females are treated as sex objects, the tendency is for them to behave as sex objects; and if males are treated as aggressive and competitive, they will behave aggressively and competitively. The teacher should stress that escaping from our pigeonholes requires that males and females perceive each other differently from the traditional stereotypes. Consequently, women will become partners and men will be able to cry.

COURTSHIP AND MARRIAGE

Someone once said that when he spends time with someone else he has given that person his most valuable possession—an irretrievable part of his life. Obviously then, dating, going steady, being engaged, and getting married represent important decisions relative to the finite time we have on this earth. These next few activities are designed to help students investigate with whom of the opposite sex they spend time and with whom they would like to interact. In short, this section presents activities related to courtship and marriage.

Computer Dating

Most students have heard of computer dating services. These services seek to match people on relevant variables: age, race, religion, interests, profession, etc. This activity, Computer Dating, requires students to create an application form which they would employ to match people for dates. All relevant options must be provided, so that rather than a question such as "What are your hobbies?," the application item might appear as follows:

Your hobbies are (check as many as is applicable):

___ 1. sports

___ 2. television

___ 3. arts and crafts

___ 4. painting

___ 5. reading

___ 6. stamp collecting

___ 7. bicycling

The following list suggests variables for students to consider:

1. race
2. religion
3. color of hair
4. body measurements
5. personality

6. hobbies
7. age
8. intelligence
9. talents
10. driver's license or not

As a follow-up to the development of the application form, students should administer the form to friends who are going steady, relatives who are engaged to be married, and married neighbors. A discussion of how couples matched (or did not match) on the variables students decided were important should result in several conclusions:

1. Some variables are more important than others.
2. Some couples exhibit complimentary traits rather than similar. For example, a wife might exhibit a need to be domineering, whereas the husband might need nurturance and desire to be dominated.
3. Some relationships seem to be inappropriate on the basis of the data collected.
4. There are other variables which weren't included but should be added to the application form.

Mate Recipe

Like Computer Dating, this experience requires students to list traits which are important for human relationships. However, in this activity, the relationship considered is the student's own, rather than an analysis of someone else's. The class is told to pretend that each student is a master chef (aprons might be brought to school from home) and that their task is to create a recipe for *their* marriage partner. The recipe should be so exact that another chef could pick it up and be able to cook the same meal (i.e., come up with the same partner who meets the description in the recipe). Some items to consider are:

1. What does this partner do with leisure time?
2. What does this partner look like?
3. What does this partner think about?
4. Where does this partner live?
5. How old is this marriage partner?
6. What kind of clothes does this partner wear?
7. What kind of friends does this partner have?
8. How intelligent is this partner?

9. Why does this partner want to marry you?
10. What kind of personality does this partner have?

The recipe might develop to be:

Ingredients: blond hair
nice smile
parents who are wealthy
neat dresser (no jeans)
tennis buff
measurements: 35–23–34
likes people

Mix With: 130 I.Q.
skimpy bikini
love for me
friends who do favors

Time: keep on ice until I'm 25 years old.

The recipes can then be discussed in small groups and the chefs could think of someone who is similar to the description in the recipe. If someone like the description can be identified, perhaps some ingredients could be added or deleted now having a real person in mind. It is important that students realize that different people like different foods (marriage partners) and that to like carrots (intelligence) more than spinach (physical appearance) is neither right nor wrong. It just *is!*

Though the recipe described relates to a marriage partner, the teacher could substitute other roles such as: father, mother, child, brother, sister, boyfriend, or girlfriend.

Marriage Vows

My father sits at night with no lights on;*
His cigarette glows in the dark.
The living room is still;
I walk by, no remark.
I tiptoe past the master bedroom door where
My mother reads her magazines.
I hear her call sweet dreams, but I forgot how to dream.

But you say it's time we moved in together:
And raised a family of our own; you and me—
Well that's the way I've always heard it should be;
You want to marry me, we'll marry.

---

* From *That's the Way I Heard It Should Be*. Copyright by Carly Simon and Jacob Brackman, 1970; published by Quackenbush Music, Ltd. Used by permission of the copyright owner.

My friends from college, they're all married now.
They have their houses and their lawns,
They have their silent noons, tearful nights, angry dawns.
Their children hate them for the things they're not;
They hate themselves for what they are—
And yet they drink, they laugh. Close the wound. Hide the scar.

But you say it's time we moved in together:
And raised a family of our own; you and me—
Well that's the way I've always heard it should be;
You want to marry me, we'll marry.

You say that we can keep our love alive
Babe, all I know is what I see—
The couples cling and claw, and drown in love's debris.
You say we'll soar like two birds through the clouds.
But soon you'll cage me on your shelf—
I'll never learn to be just me first, by myself.

Well OK, it's time we moved in together
And raised a family of our own, you and me—
Well, that's the way I've always heard it should be,
You want to marry me, we'll marry, we'll marry.

New marriage styles have been discussed elsewhere.[12] The song cited above bemoans several aspects of the traditional American marriage. After the class either listens to the song sung or reads a handout of the words to *That's the Way I Heard It Should Be,* a discussion of marriage should commence. When fifteen minutes have elapsed, students should be asked to compose the marriage vows (a la the book and film *Love Story*) they would like for their marriages. These vows should serve as marriage contracts. Several examples of marriage vows resulting from this author's use of this exercise are cited below:

1. To share and pair
   In everything we'll stick,
   'til such time that we get sick
   Another pair we will pick.

2. I take you for my wife but you are
   still a woman to me. You take me for your
   husband yet I am still a man to you.

3. Let us consider these two people joined together at this point in time knowing full well that this relationship can and will be terminated at the request of one or both parties. If termination occurs, property acquired before the relationship will go to the individual owners, property acquired after will be divided equally. Both individuals have consented not to bear children. If a child is born, it then becomes the property of the state unless one of the parties consents to care for it; with the other's approval.

4. A recipe for a happy and successful marriage includes many ingredients
and thus I will give unto you:
   3 cups of love
   2 cups of understanding
   1½ cups of patience
   ¾ cup of joy
   ½ cup of good sense of humor
   Sprinkle with sunshine and serve daily with care.
5. Together we will walk through life
   Known as either husband or wife.
   If we both grow tired of this affair,
   We'll split and never again care.

Depending on the amount of time for class sessions and the sensitivity of
the students, several role-playing weddings using marriage vows composed by
the students can be conducted.

Genetic Counseling Center

The reader will notice that this section on Courtship and Marriage has followed
the dating, mate choosing, marriage sequence. The next logical step is child
selection. This activity employs a role-playing situation in which one student
is a genetic counselor working for a Genetic Counseling Center and counsels
several prospective parents (other students) on the selection of traits for their
future children. The counselor should ask the parents such questions as the
following:

1. How intelligent do you want your child to be?
2. What sex?
3. What color hair?
4. What handicap? (Each child *must* have one.)
5. What talents?
6. How should your child look? Father or mother's nose? Chin? etc.
7. What kind of personality?

At the completion of this activity the teacher should ask for a show of hands
from those students who would have been born if such a center were in existence
when they were conceived. A discussion of the morality and ethical implications
of genetic manipulation will then prove of value.

SEXUAL BEHAVIOR

The following activities are offered as examples of learning experiences pertaining to sexual behavior. The limits of propriety, parental concern, administrative

fiat, and student interest are so varied that presentation of numerous activities related to many sexual behaviors does not seem warranted. However, the activities described, and others in this book, can be adapted to the sexual behaviors chosen by the individual teacher.

Boundary Expanding

The purpose of this introductory activity to the study of sexual behavior is to develop an appreciation for varying mores, religious and home values, and personal beliefs that result in different sexual life styles.

A handout is distributed on which appears nine dots, as shown in Fig. 6.1(a). Students are then told to draw four straight lines connecting all dots without lifting their pencils or retracing a line. The solution looks like Fig. 6.1(b). The teacher should ask whether or not students thought of going out of the boundaries (the outside dots). The relationship between unusual sexual behaviors in other cultures and within our own society—to "going out of boundaries"—should then be made. The teacher might then ask whether our society's boundaries of sexual behavior should be expanded outward (and if so, in what directions) or drawn in closer (more restrictive and prescriptive).

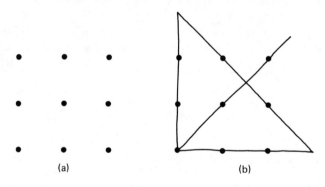

(a)   (b)

Figure 6.1

Homosexual Grid

To investigate values relative to a specific sexual behavior, a value grid might be employed. The example here pertains to homosexuality, but the teacher might substitute another sexual behavior and revise the questions appropriately. The students are told to divide a sheet of paper into 16 sections and label the columns as in Fig. 6.2.

Sixteen questions are read to the class. Each student *must* place key words from one question (and *only* one) in one square of the grid that shows how he or she feels about that question. For example, if this author were asked "How do

Very strongly	Strongly	Mildly	No opinion

Figure 6.2

you feel about student-centered health instruction?" he would place "student-centered instruction" within *any* of the four boxes under Very strongly, since this author very much favors such instruction. It should be noted that one who is very strongly opposed to student-centered health instruction would also place that item in one of the four Very strongly boxes, since the object is to identify the *degree* of feeling—not whether the feeling is positive or negative. Students may, and in fact will, change their responses from one column to another as more and more questions are read.

After the grid has been completed, have the students form groups of four and discuss why each responded as they did. This exercise gives students the opportunity to see first-hand that people's values differ relative to homosexuality (or any other sexual behavior) and to explore why these differences occur. Questions for the Homosexual Grid could be:

1. How would you feel if your close friend told you he or she was a homosexual?

2. How do you feel about two girls who greet each other with a kiss after being separated for a summer?

3. How do you feel about two boys greeting each other with a kiss after a long summer vacation?

4. How do you feel about a person who would beat up a homosexual for fun?

5. How do you feel about two girls holding hands on the way to class?

6. How do you feel about girls wearing boys clothes?

7. How do you feel about boys wearing girls clothes?

8. How do you feel about two boys holding hands on the way to class?

9. How do you feel about boys who do not like sports?

10. How do you feel about girls who do like sports?

11. How do you feel about taking group showers?

12. How do you feel about a man taking over the household chores?

13. How do you feel about a man hair dresser?

14. How do you feel about a female who becomes a lawyer?

15. How do you feel about *only* going out with a person of the opposite sex?

16. How do you feel about *only* going out with persons of the same sex?

Premarital Sexual Intercourse Scale

Another sexual behavior that might be studied in a sex and family living education class is premarital sexual intercourse. Whereas small group discussions could be used for such a study, the Premarital Sexual Intercourse Scale tends to be more motivating since discussants hold differing values relative to the topic. Students are instructed that they are to "weigh" their feelings about premarital sexual intercourse (PMI). The scale ranges from zero to 100 pounds. Those weighing a lot are indicating that they favor PMI while those weighing very few pounds are stating that they are opposed to PMI. Obviously, there are weights somewhat in the middle of the scale as well. On a sheet of paper, in *huge* numbers, the students write their weight. At the signal, the participants are asked to wander about the room, with the sheet on which their weights are written held up high, and pair off with someone whose feelings regarding PMI are different than their own. The pairs are then to discuss their thoughts and feelings about premarital sexual intercourse. Pairs can later be formed into quartets for further discussion.

FAMILY LIFE

Family life and role expectations of family members can be very satisfying and yet very bothersome. Though the home may be permeated with love, curfews, chores, and parental expectations can be viewed as troublesome to many students. The activities to follow can be employed with students to engage them in an analysis both of their own family life, and of the family life they envision when they will be parents.

Generation Gap

One may argue the existence or nonexistence of a generation gap. There are, however, differences in experiences and the ages at which those experiences first occurred. That can easily be documented. This activity serves as a means for such documentation.

Students are asked to compare their experiences with their parents' experiences via the following handout:

Place the age at which you and your parents *first* engaged in the following activities. For those you haven't done yet, estimate the age at which you will.

Activity	You	Father	Mother
Had airplane ride			
Had train ride			
A parent died			
You quit school			
Went to dentist			
Saw television			
Got a job			
Left home			
Owned a car			

This handout should be completed with the help of the students' parents and discussed during the next class meeting. Implications drawn from this chart should relate to different ages at which similar responsibilities were assumed, differences in health care between the present and when their parents were children, the mobility brought about by transportation-related technology and its effects upon family life, and other such items.

Family Values Continuum[13]

Utilizing the values clarification approach to study values related to family life can be an educationally rewarding experience. Although many of the activities described in Chapter 3 can be adapted to apply to values related to family living, the values continuum is described here by way of example. The students should be given a handout shown in Fig. 6.3.

Upon the completion of the values continuum, small groups, coeducational in nature, should be formed to discuss the answers of the respondents. The rationale behind the responses should be explored through use of clarifying questions such as, "Why do you feel that way?" It is suggested that the instructor

The following statements represent some attitudes and beliefs about the family. Place a check mark in the appropriate space, depending on whether you strongly agree with, have some agreement with, are neutral (have no opinion about), somewhat disagree with, or strongly disagree with the statement in question.

	Strongly agree	Some agreement	Neutral	Some dis-agreement	Strongly disagree
1. My family has been the most important influence in my life.					
2. My mother should work outside our home if she wants to.					
3. My father should help my Mom with the housework.					
4. The children are the most important part of the family.					
5. I have a responsibility to try to make my parents happy.					
6. I am proud of my parents as people.					
7. It is important that my parents be proud of me.					
8. Married people who do not have children are happier than those who do.					
9. What my friends think of me is more important than what my parents think of me.					

Figure 6.3

once again remind the students that there are no right or wrong answers to this exercise, and that each participant should be careful not to attempt to change another student's values, but rather better understand them.

Build-a-House[14]

Though it is useful to develop discourses in classes relative to family living, a more exotic and motivating procedure for accomplishing the same objective is the Build-a-House exercise. The class is divided into groups consisting of five members each, with a large sheet of oak tag and one color marker* per group. The teacher then reads the following directions:

> The group's task is to draw a house. Each person in the group may draw only one line at a time. You have twenty minutes to complete your task. There is to be no verbal communication from this point on.

At the conclusion of twenty minutes of house drawing, the group members write their names on the drawing and tape it on the wall. The class is allowed several minutes to wander about looking at the other drawings and then asked to stand by their own. The teacher then suggests that the drawings might be representative of the people in the group; e.g., if one group has a good basket-

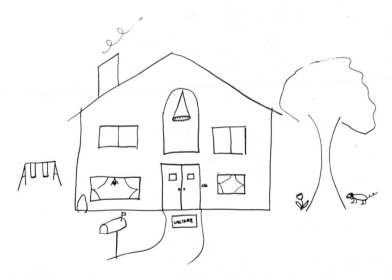

This drawing was made by a student participating in the Build a House activity. Note that smoke comes from the chimney (indicating warmth and security) and that life is depicted (pet, tree, flower, and plant in window).

---

* A pen-like coloring instrument with a felt tip.

ball player in it, that group's drawing might contain a garage with a basket attached (the directions did not state that lines drawn had to be straight lines).

Next, the students are asked to stand in front of the house in which they would most like to live. A discussion as to why students chose the house that they did will usually reveal the following:

1. Some houses were just too wild looking to be comfortable.
2. Some drawings contained people and made the house look livable.
3. Some drawings contained trees, bushes, swings, etc. that made the house seem alive.
4. Some houses had no character.
5. Some drawings reminded some students of their own house (or a friend or relative's house).

A concluding discussion concerned with the differences between a house and a home is recommended.

Family Photos

This activity, like the previous one, seeks to develop increased awareness of the family life of each of the students. These exercises are not concerned with a general, academic, safe investigation of family living; but rather a study by the student of his *own* family life.

Students are told to bring in several photographs of their family. Each photograph should include the student with at least one other family member, so that every family member is included when all the photographs are reviewed. Each student's photographs should be pasted, clipped, or stapled on one sheet of paper. Students then exchange papers and, as with Family Drawings, comment on the back of the paper about the family as a whole or about individual members. Pictures are returned to students after numerous comments have been written on the reverse side of the sheet on which they are attached, and time is provided for students to read the comments and draw conclusions and generalities from them.

Family Drawings[15]

Often children's insights into family lives are such that the roles of the family members are not clear to them. Perceptions of family life are often repressed and hidden. An activity designed to bring to the surface students' feelings about their families is one in which they draw pictures of their families in group activities or some other context. At the conclusion of this activity, drawings are exchanged among the class members until each student has had the opportunity to review each drawing. On the back of each drawing they review, students write a one-sentence comment which expresses their reaction. For ex-

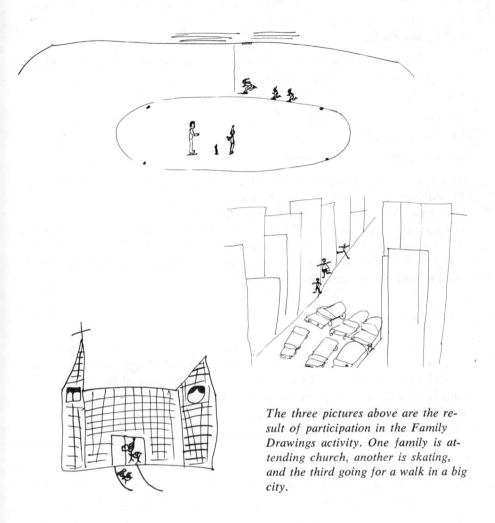

The three pictures above are the result of participation in the Family Drawings activity. One family is attending church, another is skating, and the third going for a walk in a big city.

ample, while this author was conducting this activity with a group of graduate students, one drawing consisted of a husband, wife, and two children. However, further inspection revealed the husband, wife, and one child in one grouping, with the second child off to the side. The comments of the students reflected the possibility that in this family one child tended to be excluded from family activity and decision-making. The drawer later admitted that this was, in fact, the case, and that in the future he would make an effort to include the whole family in activity and the formulation of decisions. Student comments on the back of the drawings should relate to the family as a whole (e.g., was a pet drawn as part of the family?) or to the individuals depicted. Next, drawings are returned to the artists with time provided to read the comments of their classmates.

Sibling Sequencing

Often overlooked in family living classes, but very much in the minds of psychologists, is an investigation of the relationship of birth order to behavior. To begin such a study, divide the class into three groups:

1. One group of first borns
2. One group of youngest in family
3. One group of "middle borns"

The task of each group is to list what their birth order has meant to them. Provide twenty minutes for this phase of the activity, after which the class discusses the conclusions reached by each group. A vote is taken regarding the number of students who would prefer to have been born to their family in a different birth order, and the class discusses with those who voted why they voted as they did. This activity demonstrates quite well the principle that the grass is always greener on the other side of the fence.

VALUING ACTIVITIES

Since values contribute to our choices of sexual behavior, sexuality, and family life, the use of values clarification in a sex and family living unit seems appropriate. The activities to follow are but several examples of how some of the valuing instructional strategies described in Chapter 3 can be applied to the study of sex and family living.

Values Ranking

Asking students to rank order their preferences about sex and family life will help them to identify and clarify values of which they may not have been previously aware. Some possible values groupings that can be rank ordered are:

1. A married man should be a lover.
2. A married man should be a father.
3. A married man should be a breadwinner.

1. A married woman should be a lover.
2. A married woman should be a mother.
3. A married woman should be a homemaker.

1. Don Juan
2. Romeo
3. James Bond

1. Homosexuals
2. Heterosexuals
3. Ambisexuals

Epitaph

What we value is often evident in how we prefer to be remembered. Students can be asked to write their epitaphs relative to particular sexual roles. For example, they can be asked: If you were to die today, what would you want people to remember about you as a man or woman, brother or sister, boyfriend or girlfriend? A discussion pertaining to the reasons each person wrote what they did would then be useful to demonstrate that different people often possess different values and that no one set of values is the right one.

Epitaphs need not relate to the death of the person. We all go through various stages of life and might view these *stages* we've been through as dead. Consequently, it is possible to write epitaphs for these stages of life. One way to do this is to ask students the following:

1. How do you think your sexuality will change when you are:

    30 years old _____
    45 years old _____
    70 years old _____

2. How does a girlfriend/boyfriend differ from a wife/husband?

3. How does a mother/father differ from a grandmother/grandfather?

4. How does an infant differ sexually from a teenager?

5. How does a 75-year-old heterosexual differ from a 75-year-old homosexual?

Role Trading

An excellent means of exploring values relative to sexuality is to ask students to place six sexual roles that they play on six index cards (one role per card). Some possible roles are:

boyfriend/girlfriend	brother/sister
masturbator	lover
son/daughter	heterosexual
feminist	male chauvinist
exploiter	virgin
teaser	male
female	aggressor

Each student is next told to pin on his/her chest the six cards and to wander about the classroom trying to trade one or more of the cards for a role that another student has and that he or she would like to have. However, in the fifteen minutes allotted to the trading phase, each student *must* trade at least two of his or her index cards. At the completion of the trading phase, the following questions should be considered:

1. How would you feel about giving up these roles if you really had to?

2. How would you feel about really accepting the roles others traded to you?
3. How important to you are the roles you were unwilling to trade away?
4. How well do you perform the roles you kept? How about the ones you traded away?
5. How could you better perform the roles you kept?
6. How could you better perform the roles you traded away?
7. How could you better perform the roles you received in trade?

Values Statements

Still another means of incorporating values clarification within sex and family living education is to use incomplete sentences which, when completed by the students, will indicate values. Some possible beginnings of sentences which pertain to sexual behavior appear below:

1. Promiscuity_____
2. Homosexuals_____
3. Premarital intercourse_____
4. Petting_____
5. Masturbation_____
6. Virginity_____
7. Oral-genital sex_____
8. The double standard is_____
9. If I became pregnant I_____
10. Transvestites_____

CONCLUSION

Sex and Family Living are subjects worthy of study, both academically and personally. The activities presented here demonstrate the manner in which such study can be made meaningful to students while being acceptable to parents and administrators. As previously suggested, teachers should choose those activities appropriate to their local situation, change others to make them more appropriate, and decide against the use of the rest. However, the fact that a segment of a sex and family living unit cannot be offered is no justification for discarding the whole unit.

REFERENCES

1. Barbara Trecker, "Sex Problem? They've Got a Number," *New York Post,* June 25, 1971, p. 5.

2. Ibid.

3. Hershel D. Thornburg, "A Comparative Study of Sex Information Sources," *The Journal of School Health* **42** (1972), pp. 88–91; and Hershel D. Thornburg, "Age and First Sources of Sex Information as Reported by 88 College Women," *The Journal of School Health* **40** (1970), pp. 156–158.

4. See: Henry Angelino et al., "Self-expressed First Sources of Sex Information: A Study of 266 Negro Students," *Psychological Newsletter* **9** (1958), pp. 234–237; Henry Angelino and Edmund V. Mech, "Some First Sources of Sex Information as Reported by Sixty-Seven College Women, *Journal of Psychology* **39** (1955), pp. 321–24; and Margie R. Lee, "Background Factors Related to Sex Information and Attitudes," *Journal of Educational Psychology* **43** (1952), pp. 467–485.

5. Roger W. Libby, "Washington State Board Limits Sex Education to 'The Plumbing'," *Phi Delta Kappan* **15** (1970), p. 402.

6. Barbara B. Levin et al., "A Peek at Sex Education in a Midwestern Community," *The Journal of School Health* **42** (1972), p. 463.

7. David J. Holcomb, Arthur E. Garner, and Harper F. Beaty, "Sex Education in Texas Public Schools," *The Journal of School Health* **40** (1970), pp. 563–566.

8. Carrie Lee Warren and Richard St. Pierre, "Sources and Accuracy of College Students' Sex Knowledge," *The Journal of School Health* **43** (1973), p. 589.

9. J. L. Malfetti and E. M. Eidlitz, *Perspectives on Sexuality* (New York: Holt, Rinehart, & Winston, 1972). Used by permission.

10. Nancy Adair, *A Rationale for Sex Education in the Schools,* unpublished Masters Degree project, State University of New York at Buffalo, 1974. Used by permission.

11. Betty Roszak and Theodore Roszak (editors), *Masculine/Feminine: Readings in Sexual Mythology and the Liberation of Women* (New York: Harper & Row, 1969), pp. vii–viii. Reprinted by permission.

12. Vance Packard, *The Sexual Wilderness* (New York: David McKay, 1968), pp. 459–462.

13. Obtained from William Blokker, Board of Cooperative Educational Services of Oswego County, Mexico, New York. Used by permission.

14. Adapted from Bill Blokker, "Build a House," *School Health Review* **4**, 6 (1973), p. 37. Used by permission.

15. Jerrold S. Greenberg, "Learning Games," *School Health Review* **4**, 5 (1973), p. 43. Used by permission.

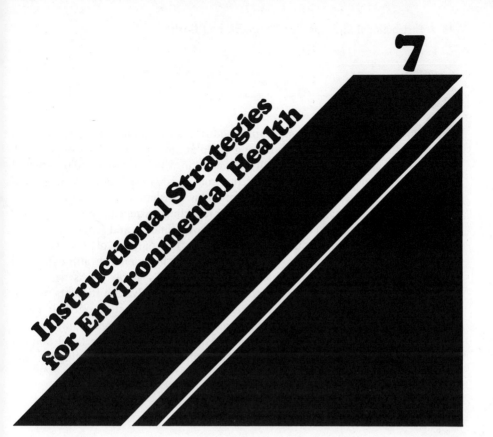

7

Instructional Strategies
for Environmental Health

One of the current, thank goodness, societal concerns relates to environmental health. With an increasing population,[1] more and more waste to process, dirty air to breath, and polluted waters in which to swim, environmental health is threatened. Several levels of our society are responding to these concerns in their unique contributory fashion—new legislation continues to be proposed, industrial firms are seeking means for recycling waste, consumers are asked to respond appropriately (e.g., keep their cars well tuned), and schools are offering environmental health education experiences. The purpose of this chapter is to present learning experiences which can make environmental health education offerings more meaningful and interesting to the pupils involved. As with other chapters in this book, a prime concern is to actively involve the students in their own learning through participation in activities requiring action on their parts. The following activities meet this criterion and exemplify the philosophy underlying this book. It should be noted that, as with other health-related content areas presented, the learning experiences described are only a sampling of what an imaginative teacher might develop and employ.

SENSORY AWARENESS

One aspect of ecological study, often overlooked in crisis-oriented health education curricula, is the sensory pleasure that can be derived from the environment. As with drug education, to emphasize negative aspects while neglecting the benefits is a skewed presentation. However, to fully appreciate the joy which can be derived from one's surroundings, one needs keen sensory awareness. This section describes learning activities which can be employed to heighten sensory awareness as it relates to the environment.

Blindfolded Activities

Though eyesight is a luxury most of us would refuse to relinquish, some experiences are more meaningful without the sense of sight interfering. In particular, where sensory awareness development is concerned, seeing distracts from an awareness of the input obtained from other senses. Consequently, this activity requires students to choose a partner and to have one of the pair blindfolded.

Once the blindfold is in place, the sighted student leads the blindfolded one on a walk around the school and, if circumstances permit, outside the school building. No verbal communication between the partners should be allowed, although they are always to remain in physical contact (hand holding, elbow leading, etc.). For the first ten minutes of the walk, the blindfolded one should concentrate on the sounds he or she hears, the next ten minutes on the smells, and the last ten minutes on feeling objects. The next class meeting should be devoted to the partner's turn to experience the blind walk. It will surprise the students that they usually miss so much of what they hear, smell, and touch.

An additional blindfolded sensory awareness developmental activity relates to the sense of taste. Students are blindfolded and seated at their desks. From edible items brought to class by each student, the teacher chooses some food for several students to taste and guess what they've just eaten. Additional foods chosen should result in the students having had the opportunity to concentrate upon and develop their sense of taste. A similar activity—touching objects or foods and then guessing what they are—can be conducted and related to the sense of touch.

Mixing Senses

Helping students to look at their environment anew can be interestingly accomplished by having them mix senses. In doing so, students will develop a greater appreciation for the uniqueness of each sense and it's contribution to the whole. Figure 7.1 provides one means of engaging students in a mixing-senses activity:[2]

Senses	Sight	Taste	Smell	Touch	Hearing
Sight		What does red taste like?	What does the sky smell like?	What do mountains feel like?	What does blue sound like?
Taste	How does sour look?		What does sweet smell like?	How does bitter feel?	What does ice cream sound like?
Smell	What does the smell of rain look like?	How does perfume taste?		What do the smells of dinner cooking feel like?	What does the smell of soap sound like?
Touch	How does soft look?	What does a rough rock taste like?	How does silky smell?		What does fur sound like?
Hearing	How does a whisper look?	What does laughing taste like?	What does barking smell like?	How does a siren feel?	

Figure 7.1

Written compositions, or discussions answering the questions in the chart, will lead students to a heightened awareness of their senses.

Zoo Tripping

One interesting place to experience stimulation of one's senses is the zoo. Since the sounds, smells, and feelings present at the zoo are not those experienced usually, one's senses tend to become used more. As with the blindfolded exercises, if students were to close their eyes for part of the visit and concentrate on one of the other senses, they would develop a greater sensory awareness than otherwise might occur. This does not mean that sight should not be utilized at the zoo; in fact, the practice of seeing and observing in a new setting is recommended. To derive even greater benefit from Zoo Tripping it is suggested that, if one is available, a petting zoo be visited so as to provide practice for increasing sensory awareness related to touching and feeling. If a zoo is not available for visit, a farm could serve the same purpose.

Snow Romping

There are many opportunities to utilize natural settings for increasing sensory awareness. An imaginative teacher will respond to the challenge of developing increased sensory awareness through use of the environment in many diverse and varied ways. One means by which the instructor might use the environment for this purpose is called Snow Romping. On a day after the snow has fallen—or as it is actually coming down—the teacher has the class members bundle up and takes them outdoors. Several activities in the snow are possible, only some of which are suggested below:

1. Catch a snowflake in your mouth. How does it taste? Feel? What does it do?
2. Catch a snowflake in your hand. What does it look like? Describe it. How does it feel?
3. Look toward the sky and let the snow fall on your face. How does it feel?
4. Pick up a handful of snow. Smell it. What does it smell like?
5. Pick up a handful of snow, being careful not to squeeze the flakes together. Place the snow between the palms of both hands, bring the hands to one ear, squeeze the snow and listen. What did the snow sound like?
6. Fall into a snow pile. What happened to you? What happened to the snow? How did it feel when you fell into the snow?
7. Listen to the snow fall. Did you hear anything?
8. Listen to the cars *swish* through the snow. What do they sound like?
9. Listen to people *slosh* through the snow. What does that sound like?
10. Act as though you are a snowflake. How does the snowflake (you) feel? Where does the snowflake want to go? From where did the snowflake come? Where will the snowflake go when the sun shines?

Other natural phenomena, such as drizzle, wind, or sun, can be similarly employed to develop increased appreciation and development of the senses.

ENVIRONMENTAL STUDY

The following activities relate to the study of varied environmental factors. Once sensory awareness has been expanded, disillusionment with the state of the environment will lead to an interest in the learning experiences described in this section.

Litter Police

A police force within the health education class could be formed to meander about the school building (cafeteria, schoolyard, etc.) and observe instances of disregard for the school environment. Mock violation tickets, accompanied by a handout defining ecological concerns and solutions to school environmental problems, could be handed to all those observed to behave in an environmentally unhealthy manner. If it can be enforced, the violation ticket might require students so cited to attend, after school (or during a study hall or lunch period), a short lecture or display further describing problems of an ecological nature. The Litter Police Force might, in addition, decide to conduct a school-wide educational program related to environmental health education. To add to the enthusiasm of the Force, unique hats could be worn by all Litter Police.

Planned City

With the notoriety associated with the development and conduct of such cities as Reston, Virginia and Columbia, Maryland, communities are increasingly setting out to develop new suburban areas rationally, rather than let them develop haphazardly. Planned cities connote conscious efforts to make sense out of a soon-to-be community. Usually a minimum amount of recreational area per resident is planned, provision is made for an industrial complex, and both purchased and rented facilities are available.

Utilizing the planned-cities concept, have the students plan a city which makes sense to *them*. By way of preparation for this activity, it is recommended that students read about existing or contemplated planned cities.[3]

Trash Treasures

To demonstrate the nature of waste and the use to which waste might be put, give students the time to wander about the school and its environs gathering objects that have been discarded. From these objects the students must create a work of art: sculpture, mosaic, or collage, for example. Those deemed by the class to be exceptionally interesting should be displayed prominently in an appropriate place within, or just outside, the school. A poster describing the work and its ingredients, as well as a short paragraph on the recycling of solid waste, should be placed alongside the Trash Treasure.

Trash Container Spying

One of the generalities about the American culture is that there tends to be a great deal of waste in everyday functioning. To evidence the truth in this criticism, and to seek means for somewhat lessening this problem, send several students to bring back to class a waste container which tends to receive a great deal of use. After spreading a protective cover on the floor in the classroom (cut-open trash container liners can be used for this purpose), empty the contents of the trash container on the floor. Wearing old pairs of gloves, students should rummage through the garbage and discuss:

1. how some of the trash could be reused,
2. how to decrease the amount of trash deposited (e.g., write on both sides of a paper), and
3. how industry might help in decreasing the amount of trash that cannot be used again.

The teacher might then suggest that students conduct a similar exercise with the trash collected from the containers in their homes, with particular attention to those located in *their* rooms.

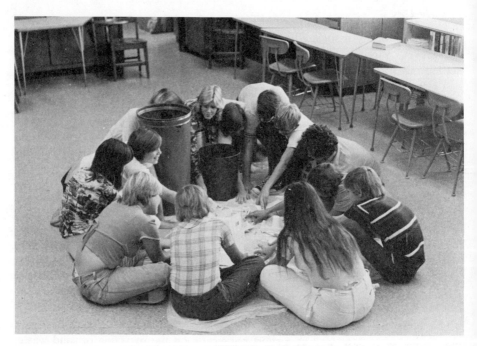

These students are enjoying the Trash Container Spying activity.

Population Growth Experiment[4]

Augment a class discussion on the population explosion by periodically halving the size of the room, which simulates doubling the population. The easiest way to do it is by using a long rope to delineate the limit of the "earth." The size can be halved at the same rate that the world population has increased and would cause the last few minutes of the period to be very hectic, leaving no time to discuss the phenomena that took place. Otherwise, the class could be roped off periodically according to convenience. The class must adapt to the changes in a variety of ways that duplicate the effects of doubling the population. For example, the decrease in amount of space per student forces many to stand, simulating moving upwards as with high-rise apartment living. Occasionally some students refuse to stay within the confines of the rope, illustrating very well that as the pressures of more people and less space build some of us want to drop out or push others out. This might be a reason for increased suicide and homicide. A short film that shows how population-doubling time is decreasing would fit in perfectly with this demonstration.

Tug-of-War

Environmental problems and solutions relate to that thin line between *freedom* to do what one wants and *responsibility* to one's fellow man. The relationship between freedom and responsibility can be demonstrated by conducting a tug-of-war. Divide the class into groups of five members each based on size; i.e., each group should have comparable strength for the tug-of-war exercise. Select two teams to oppose each other; then have each team hold on to one end of a rope and tug until one team is moved five feet toward the other team's side. If the teams have been comprised with concern for equal strength, the tug-of-war will be a grueling activity for the team members. Muscles will hurt, palms will feel uncomfortable, and frustration will be evidenced. What the students *do* with these feelings is the part of this activity that should be examined and analyzed. After the tug-of-war has ended, the class should discuss such questions as the following:

1. Why did, or didn't, you stop tugging on the rope when you started to be uncomfortable?
2. Were you afraid of the reaction of your team members if you let them down?
3. When you observed someone let go of the rope did you empathize with that person or did you deride him or her?
4. When you were close to winning or losing, did you feel that you lost your freedom to let go of the rope? Why or why not?
5. Can this exercise be generalized to any real-life situations that you recall? That you've experienced?

6. Concerning environmental problems and solutions, how do freedom and responsibility relate?

School Grounds Exploring

Many opportunities for environmental study can occur on school grounds. The following activities have been suggested by one school system:[5]

1. Emphasize the *senses*

    a) Have the students lie on their backs in the grass quietly for five minutes. What do they hear, smell, see?
    b) Have them lie on their stomachs and do the same.
    c) Use hand lenses to discover.
    d) Collect various *shades* of colors growing naturally, various colors, shapes, textures.

2. Use the *lawns*

    a) Mark off a square foot of lawn. Count the number of plants in it. How many different kinds? Compare with an equal area of sandier, poorer soil. Discuss the differences.
    b) Dig up clover roots and look for bacterial nodules.
    c) Watch an active ant hill. How do they dig the hole?
    d) Search for worm castings. How many do you find in a square yard? Discuss the important role of worms in soil formation.
    e) Are there grass, flowers, seeds?
    f) Record temperatures on various places in and on the lawn. Compare with temperatures on blacktop. Are there differences?

3. Use the *shrubbery and trees*

    a) How many different kinds of evergreens can you find?
    b) Can you find berries? What are they good for?
    c) Has anything been nibbling on, or using the leaves?
    d) How do leaves grow on a branch? Are they arranged the same?
    e) How do new leaves feel compared with old leaves?
    f) Does all bark look and feel the same? Make bark rubbings?
    g) Can you hear tree branches rubbing in the wind?
    h) Look for leaf "skeletons." Why and what do they mean?

4. Use the *buildings, walks and driveways*

    a) Look for algae and lichens growing on the bare surfaces. Why do they grow there and how?
    b) Study some ivy (a safe kind). How does it cling to the wall?
    c) Look for signs of weathering and erosion (rust, corrosion).
    d) Look at stones in a wall. Compare textures, color, shine.
    e) After a rain, find miniature deltas, rivers, valleys. See how they form.

Solid Waste Instrument Making

Since recycling has been suggested as one means of responding to the increasing production of waste products, involving students in a recycling activity seems to make sense. The following listing and illustration (Fig. 7.2) of instruments that can be made from solid waste was developed by the Wellesley, Massachusetts public school system.[6]

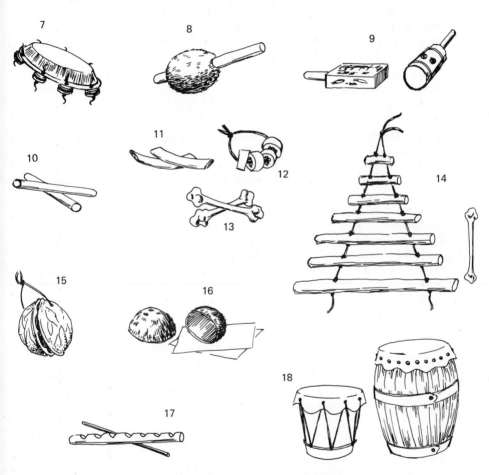

Fig. 7.2   Simple Instruments Made of Solid Waste

Water Whistle—A straw partly cut in two and bent at the cut with one end immersed in a bottle with water in it makes a musical note by gently blowing through the horizontal straw and raising and lowering the other part in the water.

Straw Oboe—A straw with one end flattened (which acts as the double reed as in an oboe) and blown into, makes a crude musical instrument. To get various notes, cut straws to different lengths.

Tuned Bottles—Arrange bottles and jugs filled with water at different levels. Tune the bottles to a scale by varying the amount of water. Mark levels so they may be tuned again easily. Play a tune by tapping or by blowing across the top.

Rubber Band-jo—Use various sizes of rubber bands (length and thickness) stretched over a cigar box or milk carton (with a rectangle cut from one side leaving ¼" margin for rigidity along either side and a wooden stick tacked across opening to brace the sides). Put eight rubber bands around the carton equally spaced. The pitch of each band may be raised or lowered by tightening or loosening the band across the opening. Tune the eight strings to a scale. Make two instruments to play duets.

Wishbone Harp—Save the wishbone from your chicken or turkey dinner for a tiny wishbone harp. String a small, thin rubber band across the opening. Wind the band over several times if necessary. Rest the open end of the wishbone on a piece of wood or empty can and pluck it gently.

Bass or Contralto Bucket—All you need is a large metal washtub, bucket or large juice can, broomstick, a length of heavy cord or venetian blind cord, and an assortment of hardware—an eye screw, two washers, and a nut. Turn the tub upside down. Drill a hole through the center large enough to fit a large screw eye. Cushion the screw with a washer and thread it through. On the inside of the bucket put on another washer and tighten with a nut. Bore a hole in the end of the broomstick or a 3' piece of doweling, and attach with wire to the rim of the bucket through which a hole has been bored. At a convenient height near top of stick, drill a hole large enough so that the cord can pass through. Tie one end of cord to screw eye. Thread other end through the hole in the stick. To play your bass, stand with one foot on bucket and hold stick with your left hand and pluck the string with your right. This will be the lowest note. To vary the sounds, hold the stick and string and move hand up and down. For the contralto bucket, hold between knees, and tilt stick and pluck string.

Panbourine—With a sharp nail, punch 6–8 holes about a rim of a tin pie pan or foil plate. Cut an equal number of 3" pieces of thin wire. For each hole you will need two metal discs—bottle tops. Remove cork or cardboard linings and punch a hole through each cap. Thread them with the wires and attach them in pairs through the holes in the pie pan. Knot the wires at each end. (Illustration 7)

Coconut Shells Shaker—Drill a hole (at least 1" in dia.) so coconut meat can be taken out. Fill with seeds, plug hole with tape and shake. (Illustration 8)

Coconut Shells Clappers—Saw a coconut in two equal halves. These are good to imitate sound of hooved animals. (Illustration 16)

Coconut Shells Scrapers—Place paper over the two coconut shells and rub together. (Sounds a little like walking through the snow.) (Illustration 16)

Walnuts Castinets—Made from perfect halves of walnuts. Drill two holes about ½" from edge of each half of the shell. (Illustration 15)

Box Shakers—Use wooden codfish box, shoe polish box, baking powder box, or oatmeal cylinder. Put a number of seeds (rice, cherry pits, for example) inside and shake. (Illustration 9)

Rhythm Sticks or Claves—Use a 6″ long piece of 1″ dia. maple or old broom handle. To play, cup one in your hand and hit it across the top with the other. (Illustration 10)

Bones—Turkey leg bones for rhythm sticks or claves. Beef ribs (minstrel bones) to click, soup bones to string and click together. (Illustrations, 11, 12, & 13)

Xylophone—Maple sticks of various lengths and diameter can be strung on a string or set on two tubes of rolled-up newspaper. For best resonance, drill holes at ⅕ distance from end of each stick. (Illustration 14)

Guiros or Notched Stick—Choose a branch or a piece of scrap wood about 1″ in dia., and 12″ to 24″ long. Whittle open notches half an inch wide, spacing them every half-inch or so. A metal tapper or chopstick produces the sound by being scraped across the notches or grooves. (Illustration 17)

Drums—Drums can be made from a variety of simple materials—nail kegs, waste baskets, flower pots, wooden chopping bowls. For the head use a calfskin, rubber inner tube, cloth which has been stretched and shellacked. Calfskin (from a drum shop) must be soaked in water 20 minutes, stretched over container and held down with upholstery tacks. Put first tack then the second on opposite side. Alternate until tacks are 1″ apart. For flower pots or other non-wood forms, use cord or leather thongs to tie the head in place. (Illustration 18)

List of Questions for Environmental Study[7]

Different techniques and methods may be employed in environmental studies. Given the broad behavioral objectives and the desired outcomes, a list of specific questions and samples will help the teacher direct the activities of his or her students for more effective learning. The list presents questions that may be completed by using the samples given on any appropriate choice which fits the particular unit with which the students are involved.

Questions	Samples
What words or ideas come to mind when I say _____?	(ecology, predator, recycle)
What do you think of when you hear the word _____?	(conservation, SST, road)
Compare two or more _____.	(animals, bones, rocks)
Contrast _____ with _____.	(topsoil-sand, frog-toad)
What are the significant similarities between _____ and _____?	(birch tree-beach tree, pen-pencil)
What are the significant differences between _____ and _____?	(trains-boats, camping-backpacking)
Differentiate between _____ and _____ _____.	(salt water-fresh water, predator-prey)
What different ways are there to solve problem X?	(air pollution, of gypsy moth)
How many kinds of problems could have arisen from situation X?	(earthquake, parking)
How many different ways can object Z be used?	(paper, glass)

Questions	Samples
How many different ways can you group these objects, words, ideas, etc.?	(rocks, bottle tops)
How many different patterns do you observe in this picture, song, etc.?	(geometric, growth)
How many different views can we anticipate in terms of this issue?	(paying the price of pollution)
How many different predictions can we make relative to X occurrence?	(algol bloom, drought)
How many different conclusions can we draw from this data?	(population statistics, rising costs)
How many different errors can we make in the process of _____?	(measuring the school yard, cost of a meal)
Given the following purpose and data, develop a plan to achieve this purpose.	(clean up litter)
Organize the following information into a meaningful report.	(data from written source or from direct experience)
Given the following items, construct a mobile, a collage, a picture, a diorama, etc.	(junk, nature specimens)
Combine the following simple machines into a complex one.	(pulley & lever)
Given the following arithmetic operations, construct a problem using all of them.	(multiplication & division, buy & selling)
Combine the following data and state the interrelationships which you perceive.	(births-deaths)
Describe the pattern you discovered in a design.	(leaves, fruit, flowers)
Analyze the given data and identify the facts and fallacies.	(toads-warts, ground hog effect on the length of winter)
Pupils view a film without sound and analyze film by providing their own dialogue. Pupils then replay film with sound to confirm analysis.	
Tape a lesson. Pupils listen and analyze their contributions and evaluate them to arrive at suggestions for improvement.	(take a tape along on nature walk)
Pupils observe and analyze artifacts.	(anything goes)
Pupils view a film and analyze film to arrive at the sequence of events shown in the film.	
Pupils view a silent demonstration and analyze to determine what they have observed.	
What are the parts of a _____?	(flower, brain)
Describe the steps or procedures needed to _____ _____?	(make a terrarium)
List the parts of X and describe how they are related.	(automobile, flower)

Questions	Samples
In solving X problem, list the steps you would take.	(snow removal)
Given the following specific situations, objects, data, etc., what *big statement can you make that applies to all?*	(food chain)
Into what kinds of groups can you place these items, objects, ideas, etc.?	(oranges, toad)
Given two or more alternatives, which one would you chose and why?	(bicycle, auto)
Given X problem and solutions 1, 2, and 3, which would you select and why?	(alternatives)
Given issue and views 1, 2, and 3, select the view you would accept. Substantiate your selection.	(pollution issues, trash)
Given the following courses of action in X situation, which one would you choose to follow? Justify your choice.	
Given the following articles reporting Z even, select the one which best describes the actual occurrence. State the reasons for your selection.	(Using Time, Life, Newsweek, etc. pick issue, i.e., SST, ABM)
Which of the following scientific inventions (X,Y,Z) was most beneficial to mankind? Why?	(airplane, DDT, Polio Vaccine)
How could we measure the size of this room? Which is the best method? Why?	(Use ruler, string, tape, etc.)
Make up a story solving a problem.	
Create or design a perfect world.	
If you were a _____, what would you do?	(rabbit, teacher, parent)
Change the story.	(Johnny Appleseed, Pilgrims)
Invent _____.	(depolluter, a new machine)
Imagine that _____, what would happen?	(world had no grass, moon is cheese)
What would happen if _____?	(your dreams came true, if you had a million dollars)
How would you feel if _____?	(your class went on a trip but, you had no permission to go, you had green hair)
What would you do if _____?	(the sun stopped shining, you were the last person on earth)
Give an imaginative account of _____.	(life of kangaroo, drop of water)
Devise a system or procedure for _____.	(taking tests, losing weight)

Town of Barnard Simulation[8]

The following simulated game was developed by the Wellesley, Massachusetts public school district. This activity presents realistic environmental concerns in microcosm format, requiring students to place themselves in decision-making roles.

Directions for the student

1. Read fact sheets about Barnard and the gift lot.
2. Decide on a role you would like to play as a citizen of Barnard. Give yourself a name, a family, a career.

    You may wish to be:

    - a Moderator, who will conduct the town meeting.
    - a professor, who teaches biology at Lafayette State College.
    - a contractor, who wants to build low income housing and housing for the elderly.
    - a game warden, who is concerned about the growing pollution problem.
    - Mrs. Nobudua, who would like to build a nature trail for nature study.
    - Mr. Dugood, a young lawyer who is politically minded.
    - Mr. Hexacre, who is concerned about housing for the growing number of retired people.
    - Mr. Goalsworthy, the high school hockey coach, who desperately desires an ice rink closer than Central City.
    - Mr. Jones, president of Barnard Trust Company.
    - a member of Barnard Rod and Gun Club.
    - a member of the Barnard Historical Society.
    - a member of the Garden Club.
    - a member of the Square Acre Country Club.
    - a member of the League of Women Voters.
    - any of the people listed on the fact sheet.
3. On the basis of the information given and your interest, how would you like to see this lot of land used? Plan to come to Town Meeting to put forth your own ideas and to justify your position on this issue.

Description (see Fig. 7.3)

1. The Town of Barnard, located twenty miles from Central City, in the county of Lafayette, in the state of Madison, has a population of 25,000 people.
2. Barnard encompasses 7,000 acres of land, of which 500 acres are warm water ponds and brooks.
3. A superhighway cuts directly through the center of the town in an east-west direction and overpasses two county highways that run in north-south directions.

4. Two main bus lines and six taxi cab companies service the town.

5. Running parallel just to the north of the superhighway is the W and B Railroad (W&BRR).

6. Many of the people in this residential community use these transportation facilities to commute to and from their place of employment in Central City and surrounding areas.

7. Barnard has an excellent centrally located shopping center, some light industry, and a growing complex of service-oriented branch offices whose main offices are in Central City.

8. There are two theaters, two bowling alleys, ten tennis courts, two private golf courses, many clubs, as well as two public beaches and a small boat launching ramp on Eagle Lake.

9. Barnard has a representative town government headed by five Selectmen elected by the voters.

10. The Selectmen appoint the Comptroller, Town Counsel, Treasurer, Tax Collector, Town Forest Commissioner, Art Commissioner, Conservation Commissioner, Historical Commissioner, Retirement Board, and Constable.

11. Elected officials include a Town Clerk, a Seven-Member School Committee, a Board of Assessors, a Board of Health, a Recreation Commissioner, a Parks and Tree Commissioner, a Board of Public Works, and a Town Moderator.

12. The Moderator appoints people to help him: the Advisory Committee, Improvement Coordinating Committee, and Industrial Development Committee, and other various ad hoc committees as needed. For Town Organization see chart.

13. There are six elementary schools of about 500 students each, two middle schools, and one comprehensive high school.

14. Lafayette State College is located in the southeast area of town.

15. A gift, a one hundred acre lot of land, has been willed to Barnard, by an old time resident, Jeremiah Dodge.

16. The acreage is situated in the northwest corner of town.

17. Approximately half the lot is made up of underdeveloped woodland, and the remainder is meadow and marshland.

18. A brook flows from the high area in the northeast corner to an eleven acre pond in the southwest corner of the lot.

19. Broken stone walls on the property and remains of a stone cellar foundation give evidence of a former farm house and barns.

20. The Moderator has called a special open Town Meeting to which all interested citizens have been invited to help decide on proposals put forth for use of this gift lot of land.

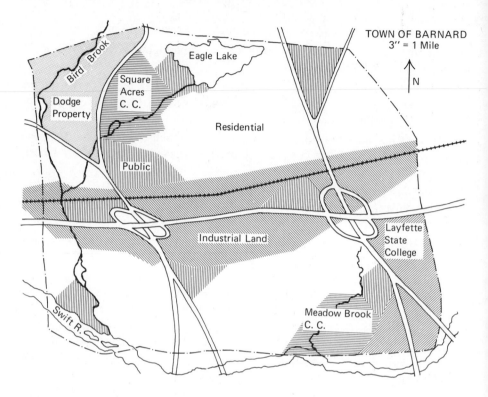

Fig. 7.3   The Town of Barnard

Barnard's town government (see Fig. 7.4)

The administrative officials of Barnard are lead by the Board of Selectman. The Selectmen act as agents of the town and meet every Monday. They represent the town and represent it before officials of the Federal, State and County governments, and the State legislature. They may, in the case of need, declare a state of emergency, at which time they are empowered to marshall all the resources of the community and take charge of all town departments to coordinate efforts in restoring conditions to normal. The five selectmen are the chief administrative officers of Barnard. They are charged in the Bylaws to "supervise all matters affecting the interests or welfare of the town," so they exercise considerable influence over town policy... The selectmen also appoint the Town Counsel, the Comptroller, the Treasurer, Tax Collector, Town Forest Committee, Art Commission, Conservation Commission, Historical Commission, Retirement Board and two Constables.

This would appear, to the casual onlooker, to constitute the power structure of Barnard. However, one must look at other officials in the town who are elected and have the power to appoint various committees. Because of the rapid growth of this town, true democracy has given way to 250 elected town meeting members. The School Committee (seven members) makes only one appointment and that

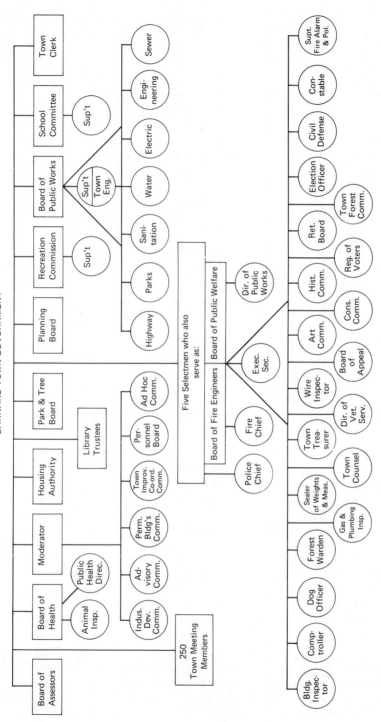

Fig. 7.4 The Barnard Town Government

is the office of Superintendent of Schools. Three people are elected to the Board of Assessors, but make no appointments. The Planning Board has five elected members and makes no appointments. Three people are elected to the Board of Health and appoint a public health director and an animal inspector. (This animal inspector should not be confused with the dog officer, who is appointed by the Selectmen.) A five-member recreation commission is elected and appoints a recreation superintendent. The Board of Public Works has three elected officials who appoint one superintendent of public works and a town engineer, and these people in turn supervise the Highway Division, Park Division, Sanitation Division, Water Division, Electric Division and Sewer Division.

The Barnard voters also elect for a one-year term a Moderator. He is elected to an unpaid position. The Moderator, by State statute, presides at town meetings and regulates the proceedings. His function is to conduct the meeting so that the *rights* of *individuals* and *minorities* to be heard are protected, and at the same time the majority is able to get action.

The Moderator's ruling on matters of parliamentary procedures is final. However, if seven or more voters immediately question his declaration of a vote, the law requires the Moderator to verify it by polling the voters or by dividing the meeting.

The Moderator is given extensive power to preserve order, including the power to order the removal and confinement of any person who persists in disorderly behavior.

The Moderator exercises great influence in Town affairs because it is his duty to make appointments to standing and special committees. The efficient operation of the Town and the direction of its development depends to a great extent on his success in selecting competent and qualified citizens to serve on these committees. He is an ex-officio member of the Town Meeting and may vote.

The Moderator has the power to appoint a fifteen-member advisory committee. Each member serves a three-year unpaid term. The terms are arranged so that one third of the membership is appointed annually. They select their own chairman.

The services of the Advisory Committee to the town are invaluable. It is required by law to consider every matter that is to be brought before a Regular or Special Town Meeting under the articles in the warrant. It consults with each Town Department, scrutinizing its budget, and sometimes modifying proposals as the individual budgets are considered with relation to the entire financial picture of the Town. It holds public meetings and sends its printed report and recommendations to all households at least seven days before Town Meeting. Reasons for the recommendations are given, and a minority report is sometimes included.

At each Town Meeting the Chairman of the Advisory Committee stands ready to give its recommendations for action on each motion that is presented.

The Advisory Committee is empowered by statute to make transfers from the Reserve Fund to provide for extraordinary and unforseen expenditures that may become necessary during the year. Thus, emergencies not contemplated at the time of the budget appropriations may be met in many cases without calling a Special Town Meeting.

The Improvements Coordinating Committee is appointed by the Moderator also. This committee was established in 1946 "to consider the planning, coordination, financing and timing of public works or improvement by the town," and to make annually a written report to the town before February 28. It is a long-range planning committee for the financing of major capital improvements wanted by the town. It does not pass on the desirability of suggested new Town capital improvements or their priority. The report of this committee is customarily filed with the report of the Advisory Committee and contemplates capital improvements in light of the Town's tax base, revenue surplus, and debt structure, and recommends to Town Meeting members methods of timing and financing construction. The committee has also general concern for the long range financial stability of the Town, particularly with the level and terms of Town debt.

The Moderator also appoints five members to the Permanent Building Committee, five members to the Personnel Board and five members to the Industrial Development Committee who guide and plan for the expansion of small industries and encourage other businesses and companies to open branches in the town. This will help alleviate the tax burden. He also may appoint special committees.

New England Town government could not possibly function effectively or as democratically as it does if it were not for the work of many hard working committees of citizens. The town creates Special Committees for a variety of purposes such as the selection of school sites, the planning and building of schools or other public buildings, and the study of special problems of concern to the Town. These committees are appointed by the Moderator.

Robert's Rules of Order

The town meeting or hearing should be conducted in an orderly fashion by the Moderator. Robert's Rules of Order should be followed particularly during the discussion and in any voting that takes place.

All members of the group have the right to express their opinion, provided that they are recognized one at a time by the Moderator and rise to address the group.

Should a member wish to make a proposal, he should place it in the form of a motion: "I move that . . .". The motion should be "seconded" by another member. The Moderator should then ask if there is any discussion, restating the motion so that it will be clear to everyone present.

A motion can be changed or amended with the permission of the person who first made the motion. This person can also withdraw his motion.

A motion can be tabled or postponed for discussion.

The Chairman or Moderator can appoint a committee to study the motion and report back to the group at a future meeting.

No other business can be taken up until some action is taken on the motion on the floor.

When voting, the majority of votes carries the motion. The Moderator usually does not vote unless there is a tie. His job is to maintain order, recognize the speakers, and see that everyone who wants to say something is given an opportunity.

CORRELATED ACTIVITIES[9]

Following are listed a variety of sample activities in different disciplines taken from many sources. They are specific, challenging, and fun to do.

Language

Compose lyrics from the sounds you can hear in the natural environment. Describe what "nature" means to you.

Write poems or descriptions about something you found on a walk.

Stop in the woods and have the group, using all senses, describe the moment verbally.

Tell stories of what was seen and listen to nature stories.

Describe the view from a given location.

As you go along, keep stopping to close your eyes and touch things—up high, on the ground, all around. Do you like how a thing feels or dislike it? When you get back, write (or tell) about how some things felt to you. Did they feel pleasant or unpleasant? Could you tell what something was just by touch?

Write or tell a story on being an apple tree for one calendar year.

Read about, write or tell a summary of the life of one of the following: skunk, woodchuck, mole, wild rabbit, field mouse, or any other animal.

Study a tree or flower closely and then write a Haiku (17 syllable Japanese verse), simple verse, short description, prose, drama.

Describe colors, textures, tastes, smells.

Describe an object while blindfolded.

Art

Take a "rainbow" trip—look for red, orange, yellow, etc. Come back and draw what is seen.

Take a discovery hike in the town forest. Sketch animal tracks located on the hike and identify. Take along paper and magic marker or crayons. As you go along notice as many colors as you can find and mark a sample of that color (or as close as you can match it) on your paper. How does texture affect the color? How many different shades of one color do you find? When you get back, make a picture, using the colors you recorded. It doesn't have to be a picture of the woods. It could be how woods make you feel.

Collect and identify seeds and make a design with different texture, color, size and shaped seeds.

Draw different clouds; identify; explain.

Make a study of a plot of land. Record changes with seasons through sketches.

Study changes in color, light and shadow due to different times of day, seasons. Sketch differences.

Make leaf, bark, etc. rubbings.

Make leaf prints in plaster of Paris. Make sand castings of cones, feathers, leaves.

Make colored sand painting.

Make a collection of leaves, soil, sand, moss to demonstrate texture, colors, sizes.

Make sketch before and after going for a nature walk. (First sketch made after talking about what might be seen. Second sketch made after walk. Compare.)

Social Studies

Find out what year your house and school were built. With other students, make a chart of how the acreage was used one year ago, four years ago, fifty and one hundred years ago. Why was the area used for its stated purpose?

Calculate the percentage of stated area which does not absorb water, due to roads, buildings.

Find out where your family's water comes from, where your sewage, trash, burnable wastes and garbage go.

What materials are used in our area for building? Why?

Look for signs of animals and birds that will tell you who inhabits the area. Where do these animals live at different times of the year? Why? Do their habits influence the balance of nature? Do other species depend on them? Do they influence man—or he them? Do they influence man's environment, or he influence theirs?

Evidence of man's effect on the environment.

Nature resources found in the area. History of the area, has it always been a forest, field, lake, etc.?

Find causes of pollution in your neighborhood and find ways to eliminate them.

Search for man-made changes and discuss whether they may be helpful in some ways and harmful in others (roads, fire break, etc.)

After rain, notice gullying, deltas, deposits of silt, pebbles, stones and "mini-geology."

Make study of gravestones for plotting epidemics.

Count tree rings and correlate with historical facts.

Determine the age of a tree and associate with period of history past or future. Tell a story that the tree might have seen in history.

Mathematics

Pace out a given distance. Compare results with others and with a standardized unit of measure.

Measure (approximately) the surface of one, average-sized leaf from a tree. Count the leaves on one branch of the same tree and estimate how many leaves on the whole tree. Then find the approximate total leaf surface on that one tree.

Select a tree and determine its age by counting branches or tree rings.

Keep weather records of temperature, precipitation, length of day, for a stated length of time.

Estimate how tall a tree is and how much it has grown each year.

Estimate height of tree (how many times taller than a member of the class).

Estimate age of live tree by counting between nodes (this works well for maples, oaks, pines).

Count tree rings and explain differences in size (due to weather conditions).

Mark out an acre, quarter acre.

Calculate the percentage of a stated area which does not absorb water due to roads, buildings, etc.

Music

Sing songs about the seasons—make up new words.

Listen to sounds of nature on walk. Sing songs about nature. Make up songs about what is heard. (Bird songs. Sounds of forest. Wind in pines, wind in hardwoods. Bug sounds. Carpenter ants, bees, etc.)

Listen carefully for a sound or series of sounds as you walk along. Put them together forming a melody or part of a melody. Maybe some of these could be transcribed and combined to make a "woods song."

Listen for insect, bird, mammal sounds, record on tape.

Use imagination to reproduce sounds, rhythms by simple instruments. Instruments could be made by children—such as sticks, shakers.

Make up a song using a nature theme.

Correlate bird songs with pictures. Also frog or insect sounds.

Science

Study pond water and identify living things.

Take and study temperature deviations in an area.

Identify animal tracks.

Plant orange, apple, grapefruit, seeds, etc. Grow new plant from parts as leaf, stem, bud.

Study weather's effect on environment.

Find evidence of erosion. Discuss ways of curtailing it.

Choose one animal and tell the kind of habitat it needs—food, shelter. Why must it live where it does?

Watch plant roots growing, test soils for chemical percentages, study different types of rocks.

Test soils for composition, acidity, etc.

VALUING ACTIVITIES[10]

An excellent means of helping students to relate health content to their own behaviors is values clarification. Environmental health seems to lend itself easily to such study. The activities below will require students to question their personal values and their own behaviors as they relate to the environment.

Baker's Dozen[11]

A means of aiding students to confront their own behavior and values relative to environmental concerns consists of asking them to list thirteen things they use which require electricity. They then are asked to cross out the three things on the list that they could most easily live without; and to circle the three things they would miss most if a power failure occurred. The students might then decide to experiment for several days with not using the three items they crossed off their list. If successful in eliminating these three items relatively painlessly, the students might select three items of the remaining twelve that would be least missed and try not using them. In any case, this exercise can demonstrate the existence of a gap between what students might profess to be environmental concerns of theirs (the wasting of our natural resources) and their own related behavior. An actual change in student behavior often results from participation in this activity. For example, students might decide to open cans manually rather than use an electric can opener.

Activities Enjoyed

As described in Chapter 3, this activity asks students to list 20 things they like to do. After this list is developed, the teacher can give the following instructions:

1. Place the letter "E" next to any activity requiring energy from outside sources.
2. Place the letter "A" next to those activities you prefer to do alone and the letter "O" next to those you prefer to do with others.
3. Place the letter "W" next to any activity that produces waste products (e.g., paper to be thrown away).
4. Place the letter "R" next to any activity that employs a reusable item.
5. Finally, place the letter "M" next to the five activities you do most often.

The following questions should then be posed by the teacher and discussed by the students:

1. Do the activities you enjoy use up our natural resources?
2. Can you use energy more efficiently by doing things with others that you presently do alone?

3. Could your activities be reorganized so as to use more materials that can be recycled and less materials that cannot?

4. Do the activities you do most often use up more or less energy than the activities you do less often?

5. How will you change your behavior, if at all, as a result of this activity?

Values Grid

Asking students to make values choices will help them to clarify their own values position. The Values Grid is one means to accomplish this end. Students are asked to draw a 16-square grid (see Fig. 3.1) with columns labeled "Very Strong," "Strong," "Mild," and "No Opinion." Sixteen statements are then read and the students are to write the key word describing each statement in a place in the grid which represents their feelings regarding the statement. Sixteen statements that relate to environmental health are (key words underlined):

1. A man drives to work in his car by himself.
2. A woman takes her own shopping bags to the market.
3. A man takes his own clothes hangers to the dry cleaner.
4. A woman uses a new can of tennis balls each set.
5. A boy uses an electric can opener to open a can of soup.
6. A woman throws a cigarette butt out of her car window.
7. An industrial company pollutes the town's river.
8. A neighbor burns his trash in his back yard.
9. A school teacher writes on one side of the paper only.
10. A man keeps writing nasty letters to the newspaper about too many pages devoted to advertising.
11. A car manufacturer makes cars that can use unleaded or leaded gasoline.
12. A mayor proposes raising taxes to install a better sewage disposal system.
13. A teenager drinks a soft drink from a nonreturnable container.
14. A man washes his clothes with detergents that include phosphates.
15. A child throws a gum wrapper in the street.
16. A mother scolds her child for spitting on the sidewalk.

A discussion of the grids should focus on the reason why certain statements elicit stronger feelings than others.

Values Quadrant

One manner of organizing environmentally related data and determining what students can do to improve the environment is to develop Values Quadrants.

Students are asked to draw a large square and divide it into four equal parts (quadrants). In one quadrant they are to list three places they frequently attend that add pollutants to the environment; in another quadrant three people they personally know who could be classified as "polluters"; in a third quadrant three places they attend which do not add pollutants to the environment; and in the last quadrant three people who are not "polluters." The following questions should then be posed and discussed:

1. What could you do to get the pollutant places to be less pollutant?
2. What could you do to get the pollutant people to be less pollutant?
3. What could you do to prevent the nonpollutant places and people from becoming polluters?
4. Who could help you accomplish 1 and 2 above?
5. Who would try to prevent you from accomplishing 1 and 2 above?
6. In which quadrant would you place yourself?
7. What have you learned as a result of this activity?

Values Voting

As with other content areas, Values Voting can be used effectively to help students explore their values related to the environment. The following questions are suggested:

1. How many of you would form a car pool to get to school?
2. How many of you walk or ride a bicycle when going short distances?
3. How many of you have ever picked up trash lying on the street?
4. How many of you would stop someone who has thrown a gum wrapper on the street and explain the harm this does?
5. How many of your family cars have been tuned up in the last six months?
6. How many of you would buy soft drinks in nonreturnable containers?
7. How many of you turn lights out when you are the last person to leave a room?
8. How many of you would be willing to separate your weekly trash into two piles—material to be recycled and material that can't?

Fantasy Questions

Often questions can be used to place students in a position requiring a values-related decision. Some of these questions, as they relate to environmental health, could be:

1. If you were the mayor, what would you do to improve our environment?

2. If you were a clean town, how would you have gotten that way?

3. If you were a polluted river, how would you sound?

4. If you were a land-fill area, how would you smell?

5. If you were a polluter, what could stop you?

6. If you were garbage, what would you want done with you?

7. If you lived in the year 2050, what would your environment be like?

Coat of Arms

Still another means of helping students to identify and publicly affirm their values relative to the environment employs the Coat of Arms activity described in Fig. 3.2. The students should be instructed the following:

In area 1 of the Coat of Arms, draw a picture which represents something with which you are very wasteful.

In area 2, draw a picture of an electric appliance you use but could probably do without.

In area 3, draw a picture of an electric appliance you use but would have great difficulty doing without.

In area 4, draw a picture of what you think to be the most important thing to do to improve the environment.

In area 5, draw picture of what one of your most wasteful friends does that makes you judge him or her wasteful.

In area 6, write what you would like people to say about you, relative to your relationship to the environment, if you were to die today.

Introspective Questions

Not all valuing activities need involve other people. Occasionally questions, introspective in nature, can be employed to help students analyze their individual behavior relative to their professed values. The following questions are but a few examples of introspective questions that may be used. An imaginative teacher will be able to develop many more.

1. How often do you use an electric can opener?

2. How often do you use an electric toothbrush?

3. Do you ask your parents or friends to drive you places that you could walk or bike to?

4. Do you turn lights off when leaving a room?

5. Do you write on both sides of a sheet of paper?

6. Do you occasionally eat left-overs for dinner?
7. Do you buy soft drinks in nonreturnable containers?

CONCLUSION

Environmental problems necessitate solutions based on knowledge and reason. Many of these solutions result in a compromise between what is practical and what is idealistic. For instance, when New York State experienced a budgetary crisis in 1976, one of the concerns was to keep as much industry in the State as possible so as to keep unemployment down. A means proposed to keep industries in New York, and to attract other companies, was to make environmental legislation less stringent. The effect of such a solution, it was hoped, would mean less expense for manufacturing firms operating in New York State, since they would have to spend less money to clean up waste products, etc. Less expense to operate in New York means that more business moves to New York, which means more jobs for New Yorkers, which means more taxes collected and fewer unemployment benefits paid out, etc. In this example, however, environmental health is sacrificed for economic well-being. Just how the environmental legislation should be changed, if at all, and the relative importance of the environment versus the pocketbook, are decisions which involve values. The activities presented in this chapter were designed to demonstrate to the health educator that such issues can be explored in an interesting and meaningful manner. Since more and more the need for these compromises will present itself, students should be prepared to analyze the stimuli for such compromise and the consequences of the proposed solutions.

REFERENCES

1. Although the *rate* of increase has slowed, the population is still increasing.
2. From *Left-Handed Teaching: Lessons in Affective Education* by Gloria A. Castillo. © 1974 by Praeger Publishers, Inc., New York. Excerpted and reprinted by permission.
3. A good booklet to write for is entitled *Audubon: Plan Digest.* It can be obtained from the New York State Urban Development Corporation, 2222 Millersport Highway, Getzville, New York 14068.
4. From CRM Books, *Instructor's Guide to Life and Health,* (New York: Random House, 1972), p. 103. Reprinted by permission.
5. Andrew Halnen, Antionette Powers, and Karen Christaldi, *Environmental Awareness Sampler* (Wellesley, Mass.: Wellesley Public School District, undated), p. 31. Used by permission.
6. Ibid., pp. 34–36.

7. Ibid., pp. 19–21.

8. Ibid., pp. 43–51.

9. Ibid., pp. 23–26.

10. An excellent source for values clarification activities related to environmental health is a kit entitled *An Introduction to Values Clarification,* prepared by the Educational and Consumer Relations Department, J. C. Penney Company, Inc., 1301 Avenue of the Americas, New York, N.Y. 10019.

11. Sidney B. Simon, Leland W. Howe, and Howard Kirschenbaum, *Values Clarification: A Handbook of Practical Strategies for Teachers and Students* (New York: Hart, 1972), pp. 383–384. Copyright 1972 by Hart Publishing Company, Inc.

Instructional Strategies for Nutrition

8

T hough often an uninteresting and tedious unit of study, nutrition education can be offered in an exciting manner. That this is possible should not be surprising. Witness the interest in weight control evidenced by the development and growth of the Weight Watchers organization, and by the quantity of sales of such books as Dr. Stillman's.[1] That people in our society are concerned with weight[2] seems obvious. That people are concerned with foods in relation to their health can also be documented. Health food faddists, health food shops, interest in books about health foods and purchase and ingestion of vitamins in large doses[3] lend credence to the claim that Americans are aware of the relationship of foods they eat to their health status.

Unfortunately, some health instructors have an uncanny knack of transposing intrinsically motivating subject matter into first-rate "yawn" material. This chapter presents instructional strategies which teachers can employ to make the study of nutrition pertinent to the students' interests.

So the study of nutrition-related educational activities begins with a concern for involving the learner in ways which relate the content to his or her life in a meaningful manner.

SOCIOLOGICAL ASPECTS OF FOODS

Though foods can, and later in this chapter will, be related to health and aesthetics, there is a sociological aspect to foods and nutrition worthy of investigation in health education classes. The United States has been described as a melting pot, since people of many ethnic, racial, and religious backgrounds comprise its population. The use of this awareness in the study of the foods generally eaten by pupils enrolled in health classes will enhance such study. In addition, the diversity in economic status of the American people means that even people from similar ethnic or religious backgrounds use different foods. This range in the ability to purchase foods should not be overlooked. Following are four activities recommended for use in the study of the sociological aspects of foods and nutrition.

Food History

There are many health-related topics which can be coordinated with other subject areas. One of these topics is nutrition. During earlier times in our country's history, foods other than those presently ingested were available and eaten regularly. For example, western Indians ate buffalo meat, and the pioneers ate fresh fish more often than today's typical urbanite. History teachers might be amenable to the coordination of colonial history, for instance, with the study of eating and food preparation; and Food History might be a means for manifesting such coordination.

The teacher should divide the class into study groups with each group assigned to a specific period of history. Suggested divisions in American history are:

1. Pre-Plymouth Rock.
2. Puritans to Revolutionary War.
3. Revolutionary War to Lincoln.
4. Lincoln to World War I.
5. World War I to Food and Drug Administration (FDA) era.
6. FDA to Present.

In addition, the teacher might want to further divide the class into geographical groups: South, Northeast, West, etc.

Each group should be responsible for developing a skit which they will present before the class. This skit should depict the food and the nutritional habits of the people in the days which fall within the group's period of history. Skits can then be combined and presented in an auditorium setting for the school, or at another school, and might be entitled "A Food History: Then and Now."

Follow-up activities might require students to develop a mimeographed booklet related to food history to be distributed in other classes; a "picture with captions" school display; or several short films of the skits with accompanying cassette tape recordings describing them.

The study of past nutritional habits and their relationship to present-day food-related behavior will provide a basis for predicting future trends related to foods and nutrition. If, as has been suggested, the purpose of the study of history is to make sense of the future through an understanding of the past, it seems worthwhile for students to examine their nutritional history as well as other aspects of their past.

Food Culturing

The melting pot concept can be employed in another manner. If students were asked to investigate their family histories, they would probably be able to identify a country or countries from which their ancestors came to the United States. These students can then be responsible for investigating the foods most common to those countries, and preparing these foods for their classmates to sample. For example, students of Italian ancestry might prepare spaghetti, those of Portuguese background might prepare a shellfish of some kind, and those from Germany might serve apfel streusel. Obviously, with such an international food feast, each student need only prepare enough food for a sampling by the others.

In addition to preparing and serving foods representative of their ancestry, students should also *briefly* describe to the class any unique aspect of the eating habits of their forebears (for instance, eating with chopsticks) and why certain foods developed to be characteristic of these people. For example, Asian Indians do not eat the sacred cow, and the weather of India is good for the inexpensive and nutritional rice crop; therefore, rice has long been a staple of that culture.

An analysis of the diets of various cultures should develop the attitude that the *form* in which nutrients are ingested varies throughout the world. However, the awareness that nutrients are needed in proper quantity, regardless of the form in which they are taken, should be an objective of Food Culturing.

Food Sociogram

In the United States, eating often assumes great social importance. In particular, the evening meal has been associated with family cohesiveness (the family that eats dinner together stays together), class snobbery (the long table with candelabra and waiters), and reward (the school athletic banquet, for example). Utilizing the unique role of the dinner meal, students can be helped to better understand the role of food in their society.

Whereas sociometric techniques have been recommended for use in schools to identify relationships between students,[4] these techniques might also be employed to create an awareness of the importance of food. Students should be asked to list the three people in the class with whom they would *most* prefer to go to an expensive restaurant. These listings should be in descending order; i.e., first choice, second choice, and third choice. Similarly, students should list three people with whom they would *least* like to go to such a restaurant. This listing should be in the same order as the previous; i.e., the least, second least, and third least they would want to eat dinner with at an expensive restaurant. However, this "least preferred" listing should be comprised only of people *who are not members of the class.* In this way, the self-concepts of class members will not be negatively affected.

The results of the listings can be placed in tabular form. Assuming, for the sake of space and brevity, that there are seven students in the class, the tables might be organized as follows:

Most Preferred

Choosers	First choice	Second choice	Third choice
John	Betty	Anita	Cindy
Frank	John	Paul	Todd
Anita	Todd	Cindy	Betty
Betty	Todd	Anita	Cindy
Cindy	Todd	Betty	Anita
Paul	John	Anita	Betty
Todd	John	Cindy	Anita

A similar table could be developed for the least preferred listing. However, since those so listed are not class members and may not be known by all students, such a table will not prove as useful as the most-preferred one. The tables are then analyzed for any commonalities or distinctions which can be noted. For example, in the most-preferred table several conclusions might be drawn:

1. John enjoys the company of females during dinner.
2. Frank enjoys the company of males during dinner.
3. Todd seems to possess some characteristic with which females enjoy being associated during dinner, since every female chose him as the one most preferred.
4. John seems to possess some characteristic with which males enjoy being associated during dinner, since every male chose him as the one most preferred.

Once such conclusions have been formulated, an analysis of the reasons behind them would help students to better perceive the social aspects of foods. For instance, why is it that John enjoys sharing his dinner with women rather than with men? What characteristics do Todd and John possess which females and males want present during dinner? Why these characteristics over some others?

Hot Dogs and Pheasants

Due to numerous reasons, none of which seem necessary to cite here, there is a wide diversity in economic wealth, or lack of it, in the United States. There are very wealthy families and individuals, whose names the reader will easily recall, and indigents of whom no one ever heard. Obviously, some families can afford any foods they desire while others can afford very little. The lesson of Hot Dogs and Pheasants is to differentiate between undernourishment (not ingesting enough food and nutrients) and malnourishment (ingesting nutrients and food in inappropriate quantities). For example, a millionaire might be malnourished because of eating too much animal fat (meat) or too little Vitamin C (citrus fruit); a welfare recipient might be undernourished because not enough food can be purchased with the dole he or she gets. The second lesson to be learned through participating in Hot Dogs and Pheasant is that inexpensive foods may possess as much nutrient value as foods costing much more money.

Divide the class into groups of five members each. Assign each group a certain sum of play money with which they are to purchase foods and prepare meals for a family of four: father, mother, fifteen year old boy, and five year old girl. The weekly food allowances might vary with the cost of living for individual communities, but the following are recommended:

1. An infinite amount of money
2. Eighty dollars
3. Sixty dollars
4. Forty dollars

5. Thirty dollars

6. Twenty dollars

Each group is then responsible for developing a nutritionally sound week's menu for the family.[5] The development of this menu will require:

1. The study of nutrients and their food sources.

2. An investigation of food prices by visiting food shops, supermarkets, fish stores, etc.

3. The study of food preparation through reading cookbooks and, perhaps, interviewing the school dietitian or cooks.

4. An investigation of recommended daily dietary allowances by sex, age, occupation, etc.

Once the menus have been planned, they should be duplicated for the students so that comparisons can be made and the objectives defined above achieved.

WEIGHT CONTROL

The emphasis upon weight control for reason of appearance and health provides an impetus for the study of nutrition which should not be overlooked by the health educator. Obesity has been identified as one of the culprits in heart disease and hypertension, as well as being considered unattractive by many. For these reasons, students are concerned with their weight status. Responsive health instructors will conduct activities to aid them in arriving at and maintaining a healthy weight. The activities in this section are designed for just such a purpose.

Alter-Egoing

Used often in group therapy sessions, the alter-ego technique allows for a third party to say *for* one of the two people engaging in a discussion what that person may be thinking or feeling but unwilling or unable to express. For example, a role-playing situation might have two students discussing busing to achieve racial integration in schools. Player A might argue that busing his or her child across town would create inconvenience for the child and A, since both would have to wake up earlier than usual. Utilizing the alter-ego opportunity, the teacher or another student might interrupt the conversation to become player A and say, "Actually, I don't want my kid going to school with those blacks who really aren't serious about getting an education anyhow." Player B then responds to A as though A had made the alter-ego statement—and the conversation continues.

Relative to nutrition (especially weight control), the teacher could establish a role-playing situation in which two or more participants discuss weight control.

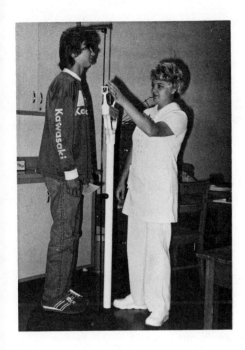

The school nurse can be an excellent aid to instruction pertaining to weight control.

One discussant should play the role of group therapist assigned the responsibility of helping the other participants lose weight. As the role-playing situation progresses, any student not assigned a role may assume the alter-ego of any discussant by standing behind him or her. When an observing student does stand behind a discussant, the conversation stops and the alter-ego speaks. After the alter-ego statement is made, the conversation picks up and relates to that statement.

This activity usually begins with some superficial statement by a discussant such as, "I know my excessive weight is unhealthy and that's why I want to lose some." Eventually an observing student will decide to alter-ego and say something like, "Actually, I can't get any dates looking like this and everyone makes fun of me." In this way the many facets of obesity and means and motivations for weight control are discussed in an interesting manner.

Problem Analyzing

The following questionnaire needs only a brief introduction. If an overweight condition is seen as a problem, students can be helped to identify those factors tending to alleviate the problem and those factors tending to worsen it. Once this analysis is made, recommendations for increasing the "alleviators" and decreasing the "worseners" can be formulated. The questionnaire which follows asks questions designed for this end and, once completed individually, should be discussed in small groups.

Problem Analysis Questionnaire*

Part I: Problem Specification

Think about the problem of obesity. Respond to each of the items as fully as needed so that other groups will be able to understand the problem.

1. We understand the problem to be specifically that:

2. The following *people* are involved in the problem:

They relate to the problem in the following manner:

3. We consider these other factors to be relevant to the problem:

4. We would choose the following aspect of the problem to be changed if it were in our power to do so (choose only one aspect):

Part II: Thrusting and Counter-Thrusting Forces

5. If we consider the present status of the problem to be a temporary balance of opposing forces, the following would be on our list of forces providing thrust toward change:

___ a. _____
___ b. _____
___ c. _____
___ d. _____
___ e. _____
___ f. _____
___ g. _____
___ h. _____

6. The following would be on our list of forces in counter-thrust to change:

___ a. _____
___ b. _____

---

* Adapted from J. William Pfeiffer and John E. Jones (Eds.), *A Handbook of Structured Experiences for Human Relations Training,* Volume II (Iowa City, Iowa: University Associates Press, 1970), pp. 83–89.

   c. _____

   d. _____

   e. _____

   f. _____

   g. _____

   h. _____

7. In the spaces to the left of the letters in item 5, quantify the forces on a range from one to five in the following manner:

   1—It has almost nothing to do with the thrust toward change in the problem.
   2—It has relatively little to do with the thrust toward change in the problem.
   3—It is of moderate importance in the thrust toward change in the problem.
   4—It is an important factor in the thrust toward change in the problem.
   5—It is a major factor in the thrust toward change in the problem.

8. Fill in the spaces in front of the letters in item 6 to quantify the forces in counter-thrust to change.

9. Diagram the forces of the thrust and counter-thrust quantified in question 7 by drawing an arrow from the corresponding degree of force to the status quo line. For example, if you considered the first on your list of forces in item 5 to be rated a 3, draw your arrow from the 3 position in the left-hand column of numbers indicating thrust up to the status quo line.

Counter-Thrust

Thrust

Part III: Strategy for Changing the Status Quo

Detail a strategy for decreasing two or more counter-thrust elements from your list from item 6.

Weight Goal Telegraming

People tend to lose sight of their goals, especially when those goals are long-term. To help students achieve their weight-related goals, whether by increasing or decreasing, the following activity is suggested: Ask students to write themselves a telegram (see Chapter 4, the Telegraming activity) on which appears the weight (more, less, or the same) that they would like to be in two months. Caution the class that these weight goals should be realistic. For instance, a loss of 100 pounds in two months might not only be unreasonable, but unhealthy. The telegrams can then be mailed to students two months hence to remind them of their goals, or they can be distributed in class.

Food Association Recalling

Though some obesity is a result of physiological factors, much overweight is a consequence of overeating. As previously described, food tends to be associated with pleasant occasions. For instance, family gatherings at a Thanksgiving Day dinner, or Christmas dinner, or Passover Seder tend to be remembered as enjoyable experiences, and may be subconsciously associated with food. Such an association, it is thought, can lead one to overeat as a reward; i.e., the food is associated with pleasure; one wants pleasure for something done well or to relieve some anxiety or frustration, so one eats food to provide such pleasure. To aid students to see food, in a conscious manner, as associated with pleasure and reward, the following activity is suggested:

Ask students to remain seated with their eyes closed. They are instructed to imagine themselves as young as they can recall. The following directions are then recited by the health instructor with pauses to allow students time to experience feelings long repressed:

1. What do you see? Objects? Furniture? People?
2. Look carefully at what you see. Notice shapes, sizes, colors, odors, sounds, voices.
3. Think of where you lived then. Smell it. Hear it. Observe it carefully.
4. Recall a Thanksgiving Day dinner there. Smell it. Taste it.
5. How do you feel? Are the memories pleasant? Is your mouth watering? Would you like to be there now?

A discussion should then be conducted which relates to the food associations the class possesses. Other holiday occasions associated with food should be discussed; as should everyday meals and the memories and feelings associated with them.

PROPER FOODS TO EAT

In addition to the sociological aspects of food and weight control concerns, health educators should be conducting experiences designed to educate students regarding the proper foods to eat. The following activities are selected for this purpose.

Food Squadron

The health instructor should be concerned with the health status of other students in the school as well as those enrolled in health education classes. One means of responding to concerns for all students relative to their food intake, requires the formation of a Food Squadron. Students in the health education class, after studying foods and nutrition, should comprise the Squadron. The function of the Food Squadron should include:

1. Observing food consumption and buying patterns in the school cafeteria and lounges.
2. Making recommendations to appropriate school personnel based on these observations.
3. Developing two mimeographed handouts to be distributed to students in the school cafeteria. One of these handouts will be given to students whose food tray evidences a healthy lunch, and will apprise them of the healthy nature of their selection. The other should be given to students whose luncheon selections are not nutritionally balanced, and it will apprise these students of that fact. Both handouts will include a description of the basic food groups as described by Jean Mayer:[6]

   Group 1: Leafy, green, and yellow vegetables.
   Group 2: Citrus fruits, tomatoes, raw cabbage, and salad greens.
   Group 3: Potatoes and other vegetables and fruits.
   Group 4: Milk and milk products.
   Group 5: Meat, fish, eggs, dried beans and peas, and nuts.
   Group 6: Bread, flour, and cereals.
   Group 7: Butter and fortified margarine.

4. Being available to instruct younger pupils, within the school or in another school, about foods and nutrition.

Eat Well Day

After the Food Squadron has been functional for a while, a school-wide Eat Well Day should be organized. If the Eat Well Day was scheduled for a Friday, Mon-

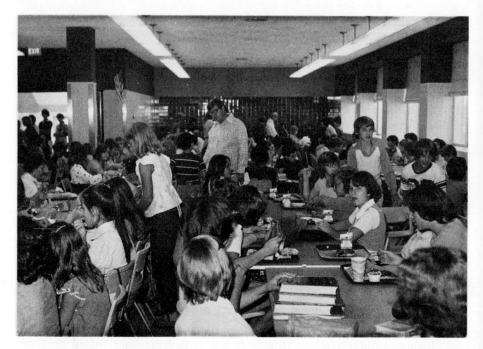

An excellent place for nutrition education—the student cafeteria.

day through Thursday could be devoted to public address announcements pertaining to the event and healthy eating practices. During the day, the Food Squadron should be available in places where foods are purchased to remind students of the day and help them select a balanced meal. The Squadron should be cautioned, however, not to coerce anyone to adopt good eating habits, but rather to attempt to educate students about such habits while they are choosing foods for lunch.

Food Investigating

There are other ways in which health educators and the students enrolled in their classes can respond to school-wide nutritional needs. Examples of these means are:

1. Students can be stationed by both students' and teachers' cafeteria cash registers and record the lunches purchased by each group. An analysis of the foods bought by students and teachers, and a comparison of the two groups relative to appropriateness of meal composition, can lead to recommendations relative to school-wide nutrition education needs and activities.

2. A sifting through food purchase requisitions completed by the school dieti-

tian can aid students in recognizing balanced meals, as well as the types of foods most preferred by the school population.[7]

3. An investigation of the refill needs of any food vending machines located on or near school grounds will tend to indicate the snack consumption habits of the school population. I refer to vending machines containing such things as milk, juice, apples, candy, soft drinks, or hot foods.

The three activities cited above will provide a picture of school-wide eating habits from which an educational program can be formulated. In this manner, the school-wide nutritional activities will be particular to the needs of the school population, rather than general in nature.

Selecting School Lunch

Since the school dietitian must select foods to comprise the school lunches sometime and somewhere, why not in the health education class with the aid of students? An activity of this nature would allow students the opportunity of observing a dietitian on the job, as well as provide the dietitian with feedback on student food likes and dislikes. The use of an overhead or opaque projector is recommended so that all students can see the lunches as they develop.

Restauranting

The school is not the only environment outside the home in which students select foods to eat. Restaurants near the school or the students' homes can be asked to provide menus which the class can use to practice selecting balanced meals. As with the school food purchases, restaurateurs can be interviewed, in class or at their establishments, relative to purchase orders. These purchase orders will indicate which foods are most often selected by the restaurant's clientele, since those foods will be the most often recorded. A comparison of any available data on differences in food selection for different meals (breakfast, lunch, and dinner) would also be valuable.

Infant's Letter

It has been said somewhere that one doesn't really learn a subject until one is required to teach it. Though originally pertaining to educators enrolled in teacher training institutions, this statement applies as well to school-aged students. To learn the role of nutrients in the body and the composition of a nutritionally balanced diet, students can pretend to be teachers of newborn babies. Rather than educate these babies personally, however, letters should be composed. These letters should specify which foods the baby should refrain from eating, and a schedule of approximate weight and height increases the baby should experience. The information included in the letter should be scientifically accurate, and so it necessitates some research on the parts of the students.

Several uses can be made of this letter once it has been composed and its content validated as factual. Some of these uses are as follows:

1. Copies can be mailed to local pediatricians and obstetricians in sufficient quantity for them to distribute to parents, or soon-to-be parents, of newborn infants.
2. Copies can be mailed to local hospitals and health clinics for distribution to parents of newborn babies.
3. Copies can be sent to homes of school children who indicate they have a new brother or sister.
4. Local newspapers can be asked to publish the letter in their Letters-to-the-Editor or health-related articles section.

Food Coaching

Since youngsters (and adults, for that matter) are often interested in athletics, the use of sport to promote the study of nutrition seems worthwhile. One means of utilizing sport in this fashion is to develop a diet for athletes of a strenuous sport; e.g., track or basketball. The diet should relate to two particular time phases; everyday meals and meals and snacks directly (several hours) before athletic competition. That protein is necessary for growth and repair of tissue, and that carbohydrates are needed for energy, are examples of considerations necessary for devising a nutritionally sound diet. Previous study of foods and nutrition will be necessary to develop appropriate diets.

After these diets have been composed, a panel of school, college, and/or professional coaches should present their views on athletic diets to the class, against which the students will validate the diets they've developed. It should be mentioned that many coaches have misconceptions about nutrition. For example, some coaches still believe that athletes should eat a steak before a strenuously competitive event, although it is known that the consumption of carbohydrates approximately four hours before such an activity is more beneficial.[8] However, even though some of the panel may present errors of fact, that in itself can be used to show how pervasive misconceptions about nutrition are, and to demonstrate the need for more research in the area.

Malnutrition Epidemic

Still another means of motivating and educating students about nutrition employs dramatization. The following handout should be distributed:

ATTENTION

This notice is to announce a serious health problem in Fantasyland. It has been determined that there exists a *malnutrition epidemic* in our kingdom. Such signs and symptoms as the following have appeared:

1. Bleeding, weak gums, and loose teeth.
2. Crooked, soft, and weak bones.
3. A lack of energy.
4. An excessively long time for tissue damage to repair.
5. A lack of usual growth.
6. Anemia.
7. Neurological disturbances.

This communique is asking for you to help save your homeland by suggesting, to our Chancellor of Health, remedies for this epidemic. Please write the Chancellor immediately.

Each student is then asked to write to Fantasyland's Chancellor of Health with recommendations for responding to the epidemic. The nutritional deficiencies represented by the signs and symptoms in the handout are listed below, and numbered to correspond with the numbering in the handout:

1. Vitamin C deficiency.
2. Vitamin D deficiency.
3. Carbohydrate deficiency.
4. Protein deficiency.
5. Mineral deficiency (in particular, selenium, molybdenum, zinc, and chlorine) and protein deficiency.
6. Iron deficiency.
7. Vitamin B_1 deficiency.

Students should recommend to the Chancellor of Health a program which specifies:

Step 1: the deficiencies evidenced by the signs and symptoms,

Step 2: the foods which can relieve these deficiencies, and

Step 3: a description, in detail, of the educational program which the Fantasyland government should finance and conduct to get the kingdom's population to eat the foods identified in Step 2.

VALUING ACTIVITIES[9]

As in other health content areas, values play a major role in determining nutritional behavior. In this section, several instructional strategies designed to help students identify and clarify their values related to choice of foods and nutritional habits are described. Osman has presented an excellent rationale for the inclusion of valuing activities in nutrition education. He wrote:[10]

Nutrition educators have done a commendable job in sorting out the reliable research and transmitting that information to their students. Some nutrition educators erroneously believe that since they have presented the facts of nutrition (especially if they have presented controversial points of view) that they have fulfilled their didactic duties.

One of the ultimate objectives of education is to be able to make intelligent decisions based upon the best knowledge available, to live in congruence with what a person knows. Syllogistic reasoning would suggest that those who know the most should behave the best. Yet the world is filled with persons who know much better than they do. The overweight dietitian knows that excessive weight is harmful to her health but she still leads a hypokinetic-high-calorie life. Such behavior could hardly be described as "rational" or "intelligent" or as the kind of behavior that characterizes truly educated people. Perhaps knowledge is not as simplistically related to attitudes and behavior as educators once thought. We need to go beyond just disseminating knowledge. Even the Basic Four and conceptual approaches have recently been criticized as being "inadequate to accomplish the desired results in nutrition education."

Facts and concepts can still leave students cold; they seem abstract and impersonal. What is needed is a personal "you-centered" approach based, in part, on the here and now of reality. The scientific approach needs to be tempered with a values-level application of the specific facts and general concepts. The values level is characterized by lifting and transforming both information and concepts to a personal "you-centered" level. This level adds meaning and relevancy to the facts, thereby increasing the possibility of their application to the student's life.

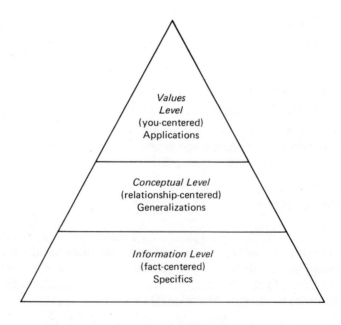

Values
Level
(you-centered)
Applications

Conceptual Level
(relationship-centered)
Generalizations

Information Level
(fact-centered)
Specifics

We need to assist students in clarifying what all the content and concepts mean to them at that point in their lives. As [the accompanying] figure suggests, facts and concepts provide a base for effective thinking, but it is our values, in the final analysis, that ultimately determine our behavior. In short, facts are needed to inform our values.

Values are like stars that guide our lives. Some people freely choose to follow certain values, others choose different (life patterns) that have meaning for their lives at that point in time.

Students should be educated as to the alternative nutritional values open to them. Students need to choose freely those nutritional values which have meaning for them at that point in their lives. Some educators, however, feel that the only values worth mentioning in a classroom are the ones that can be stamped in, indoctrinated, moralized, inculcated, or rammed down kids' throats.

Often in life, things (situations, circumstances, problems, conflicts) obfuscate or cloud our vision of the choices open to us. We can no longer see clearly those values that guide our lives. At times like this we need someone to blow away the clouds. Instead of teaching his own values, the teacher should assist students in the process of seeing and following their own values.

Values Grid

One of the variations on the Values Grid presented in Chapter 3 concerns itself with opinions and values choices and can be applied to nutrition. From responses of students on the following grid, discussions can branch off to such varied topics as how to shop wisely (both nutritionally and financially), how all family members can be involved in food selection and meal preparation, and the merits of arguments presented by health food advocates.

Ask students to mark an × to the right of each statement in the box which best expresses their opinion. After each student has done this, organize small group discussions about the topics of *how* each student responded to the statements and the *reasoning process* used to arrive at that response.

	Strongly Agree	Agree	Disagree	Strongly Disagree
Most students eat well-balanced meals.				
The majority of students spend too much money for basic foods.				
Many students know about unit pricing or practice comparison shopping.				
Most parents share information about food purchases with their teenagers.				
Students, for the most part, do appreciate the nutritional quality available through the school lunch program.				

(cont.)

	Strongly Agree	Agree	Disagree	Strongly Disagree
6. A majority of the students are familiar with the United States Department of Agriculture (USDA) food stamp program.				
7. Very few students have had any experience in judging the truthfulness of ads.				
8. Like most consumers, students are frustrated trying to get a fair deal in the marketplace.				
9. Students are usually aware of their identity as consumers.				
10. Most students drink several glasses of milk each day.				
11. Most students think about how much money they will be earning and spending on consumer goods.				
12. Students usually rely on government agencies to protect their interest in the marketplace.				
13. The majority of students take vitamin supplements.				
14. Most students believe that health foods are a good buy.				

Values Ranking

Asking students to rank order their preferences related to nutrition will help them to identify values of which they may not have previously been aware. Below appear several groupings that can be employed in this exercise:

1. taste	1. meat	1. pizza
2. texture	2. fish	2. gefilte fish
3. color	3. poultry	3. welsh rabbit
1. to be strong	1. oranges	1. eggs
2. to be slim	2. potato chips	2. milk
3. to be alert	3. yogurt	3. liver

Values List

Another valuing activity which can confront students with discrepancies between what they know is good for them and how they act is the Values List. In this exercise students are asked to list the 20 foods they eat most often. After they have listed these foods, recite the following instructions:

1. Place the letter T next to those foods that are good for your teeth, and the letter B next to those foods harmful to your teeth.
2. Place the letter C next to those foods that are good for your circulatory system and heart and the letter N next to those foods that are not.
3. Place the letter H next to those foods which are generally healthy and the letters NH next to those which are not.
4. Place the letter Y next to those five foods which you eat most often.
5. Place the letter L next to those five foods which you like the most.
6. Using only the foods on your list, compose three well-balanced meals—breakfast, lunch, and dinner.

   Then read and discuss the following questions:

1. Do you most often eat the foods which are healthy for you or those which are not?
2. Are all the nutrients included in your diet or are some missing?
3. Which foods not on your list of 20 do you think you should add?
4. Which foods on your list do you think you should eliminate?
5. How else might we analyze your list?

Values Voting[11]

A more direct manner of ascertaining students' values for group discussion is to ask students to vote *yes, no,* or *maybe* on statements which indicate values. Discussion regarding why they voted the way they did should then be conducted. Some value statements related to nutrition are:

1. People should pass a test about nutrition before being allowed to have children.
2. People should eat protein from primary sources like wheat rather than secondary sources like meat.
3. Food additives should not be allowed in foods sold at a supermarket.
4. Everyone should take vitamin C tablets daily.
5. Soft drink and candy machines should not be located on school property.
6. Everyone should have to learn about nutrition in school.
7. Everyone should become a vegetarian.

   Another means of values voting requires students to complete the following handout:

How Important Are These Food Store Factors to You?

Very important	Of some importance	Not important	Food store factors
			Low prices
			Clear and informative packages
			The chance to complain, if necessary
			An opportunity to win extra money or gifts with stamps or contests
			A pleasant attitude of store workers
			Good advertising
			Convenience foods
			Brand names

Values Questions[12]

Questions and discussion of responses to them can be a very effective way of identifying and clarifying values. Some questions which can be used for this purpose are:

1. How many of your family members regularly eat together?
2. What are the ages of the family members that eat together?
3. What are your family's favorite meals?
4. Which stores are chosen for your family's food shopping?
5. What are your family's favorite snack foods?
6. What has your grocery store done to help you make better food choices?
7. Why do you think food producers provide coupons in the mail or newspaper? Should you use these coupons?
8. What should you eat for breakfast? What *do* you eat for breakfast?
9. What snacks will you have today?
10. What do you like best about your favorite restaurant?

CONCLUSION

Nutrition education need not be dull and tedious. The activities presented in this chapter are motivating and educationally sound. These activities, through their requirement for students to be actively involved in their conduct, can result in greater learning and increased interest in foods and nutrition. It is believed that such learning and interest will result in improved nutritional behavior by students who have participated in these learning experiences.

REFERENCES

1. Irwin Maxwell Stillman and Samm Sinclair Baker, *The Doctor's Quick Weight Loss Diet* (New York: Dell, 1967).

2. Regardless of whether for aesthetic or health reasons.

3. Vitamins C and E in particular.

4. See Norman E. Gronlund, *Sociometry in the Classroom* (New York: Harper & Row, 1959).

5. Recommended Daily Dietary Allowances and nutrient value of various foods should be obtained from the National Dairy Council, 111 Canal Street, Chicago, Illinois 60606, prior to the commencement of this activity.

6. Jean Mayer, *Health* (New York: D. Van Nostrand, 1974), pp. 135–137.

7. Most school dietitians will not order foods, no matter how nutritious, that don't sell.

8. The carbohydrates will provide the energy needed for the event. The protein in a steak takes a long time to be used, and then is used for growth and repair of tissues.

9. Several of these activities appear in National Dairy Council and The Milk Foundation, Inc., *Food: A Super Natural Resource, A Values Clarification Approach To Nutrition and Consumer Education* (Chicago, Ill.: National Dairy Council, 1975). They are used here by courtesy of the National Dairy Council.

10. Jack Osman, "Teaching Nutrition With a Focus on Values," *Nutrition News* **36** (1973), p. 5. Reprinted by courtesy of the National Dairy Council.

11. *Food: A Super Natural Resource,* The National Dairy Council.

12. Ibid.

Instructional Strategies for Physical Health Education

9

The dichotomy between mind and body, too often made by some traditional health educators, is one being increasingly questioned. With a better understanding of psychosomatic illnesses, recent work with biofeedback training, scientific verification of many of the claims of the Eastern world yogis, and the suspicion that conditions previously thought of as mental illnesses may have physiological bases (e.g., schizophrenia), we are coming more and more to recognize that the mind and body affect each other in many ways not previously understood or even suspected. Unfortunately, most school curricula still separate the study of physical health from other health content areas. By way of compromise, this chapter presents activities applicable to more traditional health instruction (though still student-centered) as well as activities which pertain to less traditional physical health-related content, such as muscle relaxation, meditation, and circadian rhythms. In each case, however, the theme of this book is repeated: active involvement of the learner in the learning activity.

DISEASE BAG

The study of communicable diseases has often been conducted in such a fashion that the relationship of the diseases to the students has remained obscure. Since each student has been both a carrier and a receiver, the opportunity to relate the investigation of communicable diseases to their lives should be pursued. How to do this?

Request students to bring to class 3 × 5 index cards on which they have written the name of a communicable disease they had at some time. There should be written only one disease on each card, but each pupil should bring as many cards as needed to represent the different communicable diseases he or she has contracted. A listing of the different disease should be made and distributed to each class member, who then will be responsible for researching various related components of the disease:

1. Means of transmission.
2. Causes.
3. Signs and/or symptoms.
4. Treatment.
5. Time of incapacity.

The researching of these diseases should consist of interviewing parents who have cared for victims of the condition in question, talking with physicians, reading appropriate material, and/or students remembering the occasion on which they were afflicted with the disease.

After a week's time devoted to the research just described, the teacher should play Disease Bag with the class. All the index cards are placed in a paper bag which is shaken several times so as to mix its contents. The class is then randomly divided into two teams which compete against each other, with the team accumulating the most points the winner of the game. Alternating teams, and with each team member having a turn, the teacher reaches into the Disease Bag for a disease (index card). The student whose turn it is must provide the five researched aspects of that disease: means of transmission, causes, signs and/or symptoms, treatment, and time of incapacity. For *each* of the five aspects accurately answered (in the judgment of the teacher or a panel of student experts), the team is awarded five points. After each student has had a chance, the game is ended.

If the teacher should pull from the bag a disease on which data have already been given, that disease should be used again. In this manner, reinforcement of learning will occur through a repetition of diseases and their correlates.

SCHOOL POLICY STUDY

Although the incidence of communicable diseases has decreased with the advancement of science and the development of more and more vaccines, schools still must maintain policies and procedures regarding such diseases. Since the policies and procedures of the school relate to the diseases of *students* and *their* school, there should be a twofold interest in the content of these policies and procedures.

An activity designed to utilize student interest in their school and their diseases requires students to study school policy regarding communicable diseases. Such questions as the following should be posed and answered:

1. Which disease does the school policy refer to as communicable?
2. Who should be the school representative (or representatives) notified by a student, or his or her parents, of the occurrence of such a disease?
3. What, if any, procedures are employed by the school staff to minimize the spread of this disease to other students once it is identified in one student?
4. What relationship exists between the local health department and the school relative to preventing and responding to communicable diseases?
5. At what point in the development of the disease is a student required to leave school?
6. At what point can a student who has contracted a communicable disease return to school? Are there any special procedures for return to school to which he or she must adhere?

Numerous people might be interviewed to obtain answers to these questions: school nurse, school doctor, principal, superintendent of schools, health instructor, etc. Or these people might be asked to visit and address the class. Another procedure which could be used to answer these questions would entail the gathering and careful review of written school materials regarding communicable disease policies and procedures. If such an activity evidences the lack of appropriate written materials, the students might recommend the development of such materials to school health service personnel—or even write the school policy themselves.

SIMULATED EPIDEMIC

An interesting means of illustrating the concept of contagion has been described in the instructor's guide to a health text:[1]

> The students could act as epidemiologists in a simulated epidemic. The instructor can illustrate the concept and pattern of infection spread by applying a substance that is illuminated only under a black light on the right hand of one unknown student prior to class. (Such a substance is known as tracer powder. It is available from Ultraviolet Products, Inc., 5114 Walnut Grove, San Gabriel, California 91778.) When class has begun, ask everyone to walk around and shake hands with three people he doesn't know. The idea is to spread the substance from the original student to as many others as possible. Determine who is "infected" by shining the black light on each person's hand. Have the "non-infected" members of the class interrogate the "afflicted" members and locate the original source of infection.

HARVARD STEP TEST

Asking students to take the Harvard Step Test[2] is an excellent way of demonstrating several points about the circulatory system. It can be used to introduce pulse-taking, or to demonstrate the need for the heart to send more blood around the body during strenuous work, or to introduce the topic of physical fitness. All that is needed is an 18-inch bench or step and a wrist watch with a second-hand. The students are told to step up and down 30 times a minute. Each time the student should step all the way up on the bench with the body erect. The teacher should keep a cadence so that each student takes the same number of steps as each other student. Stepping should be done in four counts, so that the teacher's cadence should be: "Left—up—left—down." The stepping should continue for four minutes unless the student wants to stop earlier due to exhaustion. After the four minutes is up, the students should sit in a chair and have their pulses taken for 30 seconds beginning at 1, 2 and 3 minutes after the stepping ceases. It is best to pair students initially and do the exercise twice. The first time, one partner exercises and the other takes the pulse readings, and then they switch roles. After the pulse readings are recorded, a Physical Efficiency Index is computed utilizing the following formula:

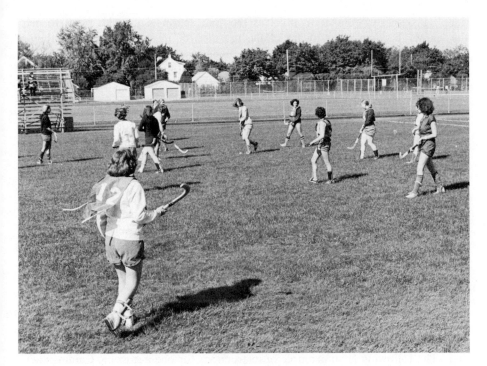

Sports activities are enjoyable ways of maintaining a healthy physical fitness level.

$$\text{PEI} = \frac{\text{Duration of exercise in seconds} \times 100}{2 \times \text{sum of pulse counts in recovery}}$$

A PEI of 60 or less indicates poor physical condition, whereas a score of 81 or higher indicates excellent physical condition.[3]

MUSCLE RELAXATION

Whereas one component of physical fitness is muscular strength, there are times when continued muscular contraction is not desirable. This type of muscular contraction is caused by stress which results in anxiety and is termed muscular tension.

Progressive Relaxation

Several ways have been suggested for the relief of muscular tension, one of which has been developed by Edmund Jacobson and is termed "progressive relaxation."[4] Progressive relaxation involves the contraction of muscles so as to help the learner become more aware of the presence of muscle tension, and then a complete relaxation (letting go) so as to experience a relaxed muscle. The following is an example of instructions the teacher could provide students to experience the progressive relaxation technique:

> Sitting in your seats with your eyes closed, extend your right arm, with the palm upward, to the right. Now make a fist and bend your arm at the elbow and contract your biceps. After 10 seconds just stop contracting all at once and the whole arm should fall to your side. Experience the muscle tension when the muscle is contracted, and the relief when it is relaxed. Learn to recognize both feelings and to be able to call upon either when desirable.

Dr. Jacobson has adapted progressive relaxation to the educational process[5] and his book describing that adaptation is recommended to teachers interested in doing further reading in this area.

Autogenic Training

Another method of muscle relaxation, "autogenic training," was developed by Dr. J. H. Schultz.[6] Autogenic training results in feelings of heaviness and warmth in the parts of the body focused on and a general relaxation of muscles in that area. The following is an example of instructions for one autogenic training exercise:

> Sitting with hands rested on your thighs (not touching each other), back straight against the chair, head hanging loosely forward, and both feet flat on the floor, close your eyes. Imagine you've just come from a long walk and you're very tired.
>
> Your legs are most tired.
>
> Feel the heaviness in your legs. They are very heavy.
>
> Just let your legs weigh themselves down.
>
> Now they are feeling very warm. Just relax them, but feel how heavy and warm they are. Enjoy this feeling. Retain it.

The whole class can participate in this activity and various parts of the body can be concentrated upon. Even the whole body can be made to relax through autogenic training.

Another means of muscular relaxation should be mentioned here just because of its notoriety. That means is biofeedback. Since biofeedback requires expensive equipment and training beyond the capacity of most school systems it will not be described here. However, the interested reader is referred to a book written by Marvin Karlins and Lewis M. Andrews, *Biofeedback: Turning on the Power of Your Mind* (New York: Lippincott, 1972).

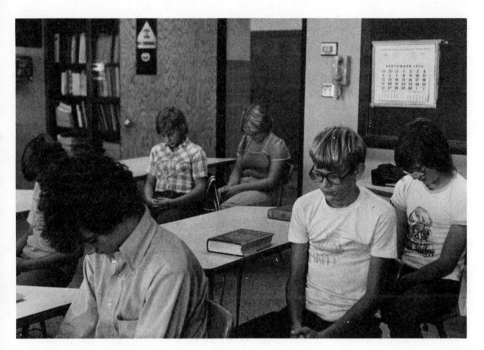

A class practices meditation.

Meditation

Still another method of muscle relaxation and stress relief is meditation. Though there are many different forms of meditation, the one whose benefits have been most validated by experimental research[7] is transcendental meditation; and consequently this is the form of meditation described here. Further, since transcendental meditators are pledged to secrecy regarding the word upon which they meditate (mantra) and the technique per se, the method described here is a combination of the relaxation response described by Benson[8] and his colleagues and transcendental meditation. The relaxation response is the name coined to describe the physiological reactions of the body to meditation. These reactions include decreased body metabolism, lowered heart rate, lowered respiratory rate, and muscle relaxation. In fact, the relaxation response is described as just the opposite of the much publicized fight-or-flight reaction.

To obtain the relaxation response students should be told to sit quietly with their backs against an upright chair, their feet on the floor, and their eyes closed. This position is similar to that prescribed for autogenic training. While keeping this position for 20 minutes, students should be repeating the same word (e.g., calm) over and over again. When students realize that other thoughts have en-

tered their minds they should return to the word being repeated. It is recommended that to be most effective this meditative process not be attempted shortly
after eating, and should be repeated twice daily (once in the morning and once
before dinner). A discussion with the class regarding their subjective experience
of the relaxation response and a physiological explanation of what has occurred
will interest students in physical health.

SLEEP STUDY

Though health educators verbalize the importance of sleep, little if any significant
part of a unit on physical health is devoted to this subject. It is true that sleep is
an area of investigation in which many questions remain unanswered. However,
it is not generally known how much we do know about sleep. For instance, it is
known that, for youth, sleep is associated with the release of the growth hormone
(Luteinizing Hormone); and with the secretion of Testosterone in males during
puberty. It is known that during sleep: the high level of hormonal secretions aids
cell division, thus restoring worn tissue; cells of the skin multiply twice as fast;
and the heartbeat rate slows, thereby affording the heart muscle a rest. Sleep is
also associated with psychological wellness (e.g., it reduces irritability).[9]

It is further recognized that sleep occurs more readily under some conditions
than others. It is suggested that one sleep in a familiar and comfortable environment that is quiet and of moderate temperature; that this environment contain
little lighting, be well ventilated, and be nonodorous; and that the sleeper wear
loose-fitting clothing, use blankets of light weight, and refrain from the ingestion
of stimulants prior to sleep (e.g., caffeine).

With such knowledge, health educators should be concerned with helping
their students obtain good sleep and the benefits thereof. The accompanying chart
has been successfully used with students to investigate the effects of their sleeping
behavior.

Daily Sleep Chart[10]

Name _____   Monday's date _____

	Mon.	Tues.	Wed.	Thurs.	Fri.	Sat.	Sun.
1. Time to sleep	1.	1.	1.	1.	1.	1.	1.
2. Time woke up	2.	2.	2.	2.	2.	2.	2.
Hours of sleep	___ hrs.	___ hrs.	___ hrs.	___ hrs.	___ hrs.	___ hrs.	___ hrs.
Check one: When woke up							
1. Felt tired	1. ___	1. ___	1. ___	1. ___	1. ___	1. ___	1. ___
2. OK	2. ___	2. ___	2. ___	2. ___	2. ___	2. ___	2. ___
3. Felt great	3. ___	3. ___	3. ___	3. ___	3. ___	3. ___	3. ___

Check Those Spaces That Apply:

Conditions	Mon.	Tues.	Wed.	Thurs.	Fri.	Sat.	Sun.
1. Temperature (hot, cold, ok)							
2. Too noisy							
3. Too much light							
4. Ate before going to bed							
5. Restful time before bed							
6. Tight night clothes							
7. Could hear TV							
8. Plenty of fresh air							
9. Awoken by noise or person							
10. Drank coffee or cola before bed							

When the responses on this chart were analyzed, it was concluded that long sleepers (more than 10 hours) profited more from their sleep than did short sleepers (less than 7½ hours).

Results of Sleep Charting

	Felt Tired	OK	Felt Great
long sleepers	1 student	10 students	7 students
short sleepers	10 students	4 students	1 student

Relaxation exercises (progressive relaxation, autogenic training, or meditation) can then be practiced by students as aids to initiating sleep and eliminating feelings of sleeplessness.

DENTAL HEALTH

The following dental health education activities were written to be utilized in a student-centered classroom situation and require minimum, if any, teacher interpretation and direction. Each activity was worded as it could appear on an activity card to be available to be used by the student in a self-instructional set-

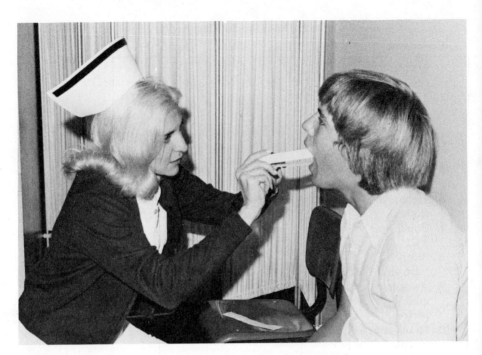

The school nurse can be an excellent resource person and a help to the health educator.

ting. Of course, activities may need to be rewritten as the teacher considers the specifics of his or her own temperament, students, circumstances, and expectations.

1. Collect and construct a bulletin board of dental products and/or advertisements of dental products.
2. How much did you eat yesterday? Make a list of all the food you ate yesterday. Using the nutrition books in the classroom, look up the sugar content in each of the foods on your list. For some of the foods, you may have to note approximate measures. Measure out the total amount of sugar you ate and put it into a bottle labeled with your name. Many chances for tooth damage?
3. Set up a "Dental Care" supply counter. Role-play a shopping trip to purchase a toothbrush, a tube of toothpaste, and a package of dental floss. Do you know all the facts you need to know to make wise selections? If not, ask the teacher.
4. Prepare pictures, posters, and/or collages re: importance of brushing and flossing, flossing and brushing techniques, good nutrition, visiting your dentist.
5. Construct a chain of decay. Each factor that contributes to the decay process can be written or pictured on an individual link made of construction paper.

Other pictures or words can be added to show how each link can be broken to limit decay.

6. Construct a calendar. Make the picture for each month pertain to dental health. (This would make a nice gift for someone.)

7. Write a TV commercial or short play recommending periodic professional dental exams.

8. Make up your own "Dental Health Dictionary." Record and define (using texts in the classroom) any word new to you connected with teeth, mouth, nutrition, general health. From all of the class dictionaries, we will compile a "Dental Health Dictionary" to be placed in our school library.

9. Prepare a dental-health quiz and interview several adults to determine ideas people have about modern dental health.

10. Design a bulletin board of snack foods (fruits, raw vegetables, nuts, milk, juices, etc.) to substitute for the usual sweet snacks.

11. Plan and have a party, using such snacks as fresh fruits, dried fruits, raw vegetables, juices, milk punches, etc., instead of the usual party foods.

*12. Out of toothpaste? Mix your own: Combine equal parts of finely-powdered table salt and baking soda. Add a few drops of peppermint flavoring, if available.

13. Construct a traveling "Dental Health Wagon" to carry dental health messages to other classes, other schools. Decide how you are going to present these messages. Some suggestions include plays, puppet shows, demonstrations.

GENETIC COUNSELING

The alter-ego technique is an excellent means of introducing the topic of genetic counseling and inherited diseases. Distribute the following role-playing descriptions on index cards to students who will be acting these parts:

Betty: You are a young black woman, age 24. You come from a large family and have always wanted three children. You married Tom three years ago when you both agreed that children were a vital ingredient of a good marriage. You have sickle-cell trait but never knew it until just now.

Tom: You are a young black man, age 26. You love your wife, Betty, and want all her life's desires to be fulfilled. You love children in general and want to have three. You are active in social issues, and believe that liberalized abortion and attempts at population control are means devised by those wishing to limit the number of blacks in the United States. You have sickle-cell trait but never knew it until now.

Dr. Thomas: You are a white physician who is in the process of explaining to Betty and Tom the implications of a husband and wife who both have sickle-cell trait having children.

Mr. Gray: You are the town's Director of Social Services. In that role you supervise medicaid, medicare, and welfare departments. You were brought to this town because the taxpayers wanted fewer people to need social services, thereby decreasing their tax payments.

The students should then be asked to imagine that Betty and Tom are in a meeting with Dr. Thomas and Mr. Gray at which time they are to be told about their sickle-cell trait, implications of this condition, and the town's desire that they not conceive children. Betty and Tom should explain their wishes, and present their arguments for having children in spite of the fact that they both have sickle-cell trait. At any time, another student can kneel behind any of the role players and speak for that person. The one kneeling will be the alter ego of the role player, expressing what he or she believes is not being said but is being felt by that role player. At the conclusion of the role-playing incident, the class will vote whether they think Betty and Tom should conceive children or not.

Several topics, which will result in much learning, may be presented during this activity:

1. Sickle-cell disease
2. Abortion
3. Genetic counseling
4. Adoption
5. Social and personal responsibility
6. Amniocentesis

and much learning will result.

MAD SCIENTIST

An ingenious teacher can develop a not-so-spectacular activity into one that will long be remembered by each student. An example of this is the teacher who can, with a little Shakespeare within, help students to behave as mad scientists. Simple experiments can be used for this purpose, two of which are described below, but the important aspect of this activity is the zaniness underlying it. Students should be asked to wear long shirts, smocks, raincoats, or whatever can serve as a laboratory coat. In addition, students should be encouraged to bring in any accoutrements such as white cotton balls for gray hair or toy eyeglasses. Some students will walk with a limp while others will talk with an accent. In any case, most will have fun and, if the experiments are organized properly, much learning will occur.

An experiment which can be used in the mad scientist activity is one in which each student inoculates petri dishes from swabs from various areas of his/her body (throat, ears, etc.).[11] The dish is then placed in a warm area and, if an uninoculated dish is placed alongside, the bacterial growth can be clearly observed after several days.

Another experiment that illustrates the importance of proper food handling[12] can be conducted by boiling peeled potatoes and inoculating them with microorganisms by touching them with dirty hands or utensils. Then place the potatoes in sterile containers, keep the containers in a warm place, and observe the growth of microorganisms. Uninoculated potatoes should be used as a sterile control.

SENSE APPRECIATION

One aspect of physical health often overlooked in health education curricula is the development of the appreciation of one's senses. The best way to accomplish this objective is to require students to concentrate on one sense, or eliminate one sense so as to appreciate its importance. There are several ways to do this, some of which follow:

1. Have students close their eyes, place their extended arms out to their sides and then, by bending the elbows, touch the tips of their noses.
2. Have students close their eyes, taste various foods, and guess what they just tasted.
3. Play pin the tail on the donkey.
4. Have students bend down to pick something up while standing on one foot only.
5. Have students close their eyes, feel some object, and guess what they just felt.
6. Open the windows of the classroom, then have the students close their eyes and listen to and identify as many different sounds as they can.

SPYING

A simple activity to help students learn factual information about physical health requires them to be observant as spies. Divide the class into teams of three members each. Give each team a chance to view a collage developed by the teacher upon which appears sentences, objects, pictures, etc. that relate some piece of information about physical health. After the groups have looked at the collage for three minutes, it should be put away. The teams are then asked to compile a list of sentences that pertain to physical health and that could be inferred from the collage. The team with the most sentences that can be related to something appearing on the collage is the winner. It is important that when this game is introduced, the theme of the collage *not* be identified. In other words, students should not be told that they will have to write sentences pertaining to physical health. Rather they should be told to be observant as spies and to try to create an accurate picture of the collage in their minds. With a little bit of a theatrical introduction by the teacher, this activity will motivate students to remember factual information about the topic on which the collage is focused.

CIRCADIAN RHYTHMING

It is known that some are "night people" and others "day people." For most people, changes in energy levels, temperature, and hormone levels occur at predictable times during each day. The body has its own daily cycles and rhythm. This has been termed "circadian rhythm." Breathing through the nose is an example of a body rhythm that is somewhat regular. It has been found that when breathing through the nose there is an involuntary back-and-forth shifting between left and right nostrils at three hour intervals.[13] Keeping track of circadian rhythms, or body charting, will help students to learn about this phenomenon as well as to relate it to their own bodies. The following chart should be kept daily for one week and analyzed by students at that time:

Circadian Rhythm Chart*

Time: For the 24 hour period   from _____ to _____

A. *Sleep and Napping*

    1. When did you go to bed?   _____

    2. How long did it take you to fall asleep?   _____

    3. Did you sleep well?   _____

    4. When did you wake up?   _____

    5. Did you use an alarm?   _____

    6. Did you feel alert?   _____

    7. Did you take any naps? If so, when?_____

B. *Appetite and Eating*

    8. At what times did you experience hunger pangs?   _____

    9. When did you have breakfast?   _____

                      Lunch?   _____

                      Dinner?   _____

   10. Which meal did you like best?   _____

---

* Adapted from Marvin Karlins and Lewis M. Andrews, *Biofeedback: Turning On the Power of Your Mind*, pp. 104–105. Copyright © 1972 by Marvin Karlins and Lewis M. Andrews. Reproduced by permission of J. B. Lippincott Company.

11. When did you snack? _____
12. Total number of snacks? _____
13. How did you eat during the last 24
    hours? (Check one) _____No appetite
    _____As usual
    _____Glutton

C. *Health*

14. Weight before breakfast? _____
15. Time of bowel movements? _____
16. Nature of bowel movements? (Nor-
    mal, constipated, diarrhea) _____
17. Any health related symptoms? If so,_____
    when and what? _____

D. *Activity*

18. Type of sexual activity (E.g., none,
    masturbation, petting, etc.) during
    this 24 hour period. _____
19. When? _____
20. Type of physical exercise during this
    24 hour period? _____
21. When? _____
22. On the whole, how would you de-
    scribe yourself during the last 24
    hours? _____Clumsy
    _____Normal
    _____Adroit

E. *Moods*

23. At what time did you feel:
    alert? _____
    tired? _____
    productive? _____
    mentally dull? _____
    athletic? _____
    agitated? _____
    happy? _____
    depressed? _____
    sensitive? _____
    disoriented? _____
24. At what times did you feel like a
    smoke, drug, or some relief? _____
25. Did you have any good fantasies? _____
26. When? _____
27. Did you have any bad fantasies? _____
28. When?

(Cont.)

29. On the whole, when could you concentrate easily? _____
    When were you easily distracted? _____
    When did you feel normal? _____
30. Were you more introverted or extroverted, and when? _____
31. How would you summarize your mood during the last 24 hours? (Happy, sad, despondent, etc.) _____

To analyze this chart, students should look for obvious rhythms (e.g., every other day they classify as "happy") whether on a daily or other cycle. They should then be asked to infer from their chart the implications for their behavior. For example, a student who wants to lose weight might arrange to be physically active at the time during each day that he or she would expect to feel hunger pangs. In any case, body rhythm charting is interesting and educational, and relates *directly* to each and every student.

SAFETY EDUCATION

As shown in Tables 9.1 and 9.2, accidents can be quite serious. To study means of preventing such accidents (i.e., safety education), the following learning experiences are recommended.

School Safety Investigation

A study of the incidence of accidents in school and on school grounds (playground, athletic field, etc.) can be conducted. Such a study will reveal those places most conducive to accidents, and provide insight into means of preventing such mishaps. For instance, if accidents have occurred frequently in the gymnasium, a program to prevent school accidents might result in:

1. padding of gymnasium walls,

2. replacing of obsolete equipment, and

3. development of a Leader's Squad consisting of athletically skilled youngsters trained to recognize dangerous situations and to quickly eliminate the danger.

Indications of places in the school and on school grounds where accidents are likely can be obtained through careful review of accident reports kept in school files. Most schools require such reports to be completed by either the school staff member first responding to an injured student or by the school personnel responsible for that area (e.g., the physical education teacher who was teaching the class in the gymnasium when a student was injured). The results of this procedure might be surprising to some students when in-school accidents are compared to out-of-school accidents (see Tables 9.3 and 9.4).

Table 9.1

Accidental Deaths by Age, Sex, and Type[14]

(Data are official figures for 1970)

Age and Sex	ALL TYPES	Motor-Vehicle	Falls	Drowning†	Fires, Burns	Ingest. of Food, Object	Fire-arms	Poison (solid, liquid)	Poison by Gas	% Male All Types
All Ages	114,638	54,633	16,926	7,860	6,718	2,753	2,406	3,679	1,620	70%
Under 5	6,594	1,915	340	890	848	906	93	228	34	58%
5 to 14	8,203	4,159	198	1,550	609	122	413	44	58	69%
15 to 24	24,336	16,720	425	2,330	385	166	728	1,010	384	80%
25 to 34	12,842	7,886	391	810	437	133	377	677	242	80%
35 to 44	11,137	5,760	720	710	566	195	272	517	231	77%
45 to 54	12,415	5,913	1,163	660	889	303	230	488	250	73%
55 to 64	11,749	5,186	1,679	460	943	315	174	355	200	72%
65 to 74	10,644	4,084	2,565	280	951	280	75	210	123	63%
75 & over	16,624	3,179	9,444	150	1,077	333	46	153	96	46%
Age unknown	94	31	3	20	13	0	0	1	2	78%
Sex										
Male	79,756	39,274	8,734	6,673	3,988	1,654	2,060	2,369	1,193	
Female	34,882	15,359	8,192	1,187	2,730	1,099	346	1,310	427	
Percent male	70%	72%	52%	85%	59%	60%	86%	60%	74%	

Table 9.2
Accidents and Other Causes of Death[15]

Cause	Number of Deaths			Death Rates*		
	Total	Male	Female	Total	Male	Female
All Ages						
All Causes · · · · · · · · · · · · · · ·	1,921,031	1,078,478	842,553	942.6	1,087.1	805.4
Heart disease · · · · · · · · · · ·	735,542	417,918	317,624	380.9	421.3	303.6
Cancer · · · · · · · · · · · · · · ·	330,730	180,157	150,573	162.3	181.6	143.9
Stroke (cerebrovascular disease) · · · ·	207,168	93,456	113,710	101.6	94.2	108.7
Accidents · · · · · · · · · · · · · · ·	114,638	79,755	34,882	56.2	80.4	33.3
Motor-vehicle · · · · · · · · ·	54,633	39,274	15,359	28.8	39.6	14.7
Falls · · · · · · · · · · · · ·	16,928	8,734	8,192	8.3	8.8	7.8
Drowning · · · · · · · · · ·	7,860	6,673	1,187	3.9	6.7	1.1
Fires, burns · · · · · · · ·	6,718	3,988	2,730	3.3	4.0	2.6
Poison (solid, liquid) · · · ·	3,679	2,369	1,310	1.8	2.4	1.3
Pneumonia · · · · · · · · · · ·	59,032	33,261	25,771	29.0	33.5	24.6
Diabetes mellitus · · · · · · · ·	38,324	15,715	22,609	18.8	15.8	21.6
Arteriosclerosis · · · · · · · ·	31,882	13,767	17,915	15.5	13.9	17.1
Cirrhosis of liver · · · · · · · ·	31,399	20,382	11,017	15.4	20.5	10.5
Suicide · · · · · · · · · · · ·	23,480	16,629	6,851	11.5	16.8	6.5
Homicide · · · · · · · · · · ·	16,848	13,278	3,570	8.3	13.4	3.4
Congenital anomalies · · · · · · · ·	16,824	8,907	7,917	8.3	9.0	7.6
1 to 14 Years						
All causes · · · · · · · · · · · · ·	28,395	16,985	11,410	52.2	61.3	42.8
Accidents · · · · · · · · · · ·	12,503	8,259	4,244	23.0	29.8	15.9
Motor-vehicle · · · · · · · · ·	5,731	3,616	2,115	10.5	13.1	7.9
Drowning · · · · · · · · ·	2,350†	1,770†	580†	4.3	6.4	2.2
Fires, burns · · · · · · · ·	1,322	731	591	2.4	2.6	2.2
Firearms · · · · · · · ·	502	401	101	0.9	1.4	0.4

Cause						
Cancer	3,456	1,967	1,489	6.4	7.1	5.0
Congenital anomalies	2,232	1,175	1,057	4.1	4.2	4.0
Pneumonia	1,623	889	734	3.0	3.2	2.8
Homicide	618	345	273	1.1	1.2	1.0
Heart disease	581	311	270	1.1	1.1	1.0
Stroke (cerebrovascular disease)	403	242	261	0.7	0.9	1.0

15 to 24 Years

Cause						
All causes	45,281	33,076	12,185	126.5	186.8	67.5
Accidents	24,336	19,396	4,940	68.0	109.4	27.4
Motor-vehicle	16,720	12,855	3,865	46.7	72.5	21.4
Drowning	2,330†	2,140†	190†	6.5	12.1	1.1
Poison (solid, liquid)	1,010	818	192	2.8	4.6	1.1
Firearms	726	846	80	2.0	3.6	0.4
Homicide	4,157	3,333	824	11.6	18.8	4.6
Suicide	3,128	2,378	750	8.7	13.4	4.2
Cancer	2,931	1,817	1,114	8.2	10.3	6.2
Heart disease	1,054	642	412	2.9	3.6	2.3

75 Years and Over

Cause						
All Causes	737,477	341,006	396,471	9,706.2	11,571.3	8,522.6
Heart disease	344,824	156,297	188,527	4,538.4	5,303.6	4,052.6
Stroke (cerebrovascular disease)	122,338	48,902	73,436	1,610.1	1,659.4	1,578.6
Cancer	91,556	48,059	43,497	1,205.0	1,630.8	935.0
Pneumonia	27,353	13,645	13,708	360.0	463.0	294.7
Arteriosclerosis	25,412	10,231	15,181	334.5	347.2	326.3
Accidents	16,718	7,761	8,957	220.0	263.4	192.5
Falls	9,447	3,615	5,932	124.3	119.3	127.5
Motor-vehicle	3,210	2,026	1,184	42.2	68.7	25.5
Fires, burns	1,090	526	584	14.3	17.8	12.1
Surgical complications	989	517	472	13.0	17.5	10.1
Diabetes mellitus	14,916	5,334	9,582	196.3	181.0	206.0
Emphysema	7,314	6,122	1,192	96.3	207.7	25.6

† Partly estimated.   * Deaths per 100,000 population.

Table 9.3*
Injuries to School-Age
Children by Location

Location	Percent
School buildings	24
School grounds	28
On way to and from school	5
Home	20
Other	23

* C. L. Anderson, *School Health Practice,* 5th edition (St. Louis: The C. V. Mosby Co., 1968), p. 171. Used by permission.

Table 9.4*
Injury Rates by Location and Grade Level (per 100,000 Students)

Grade	All injury rate	School building	School grounds	Going to or from school	Home	Other
Kindergarten to 3	11.2	1.4	3.4	0.8	3.5	2.1
4 to 6	16.3	2.4	5.4	1.0	3.6	3.9
7 to 9	23.7	7.8	5.5	1.0	3.5	5.9
10 to 12	24.1	9.0	7.1	0.6	2.2	5.2
All grades	16.6	4.0	4.7	0.8	3.3	3.8

* *Ibid.,* p. 172.

Cornering

Instead of discussing accident-prone behavior, students can view it for themselves. Students can be allowed to stand at the corner of a busy intersection near the school and observe traffic patterns, pedestrian behavior, bicycling norms, etc. A written record of the unsafe behavior observed can enrich a subsequent discussion on safety. If videotaping or film-making equipment is available, the recording and later play back of unsafe behavior can provide a real-life situation for analysis.

Bicycle Gang

Students who own and ride bicycles can form a bicycle gang similar to a motorcycle gang. An insignia can be drawn or tie-dyed on tee shirts worn by the gang.

Bicycling safety activities can be organized, of which the following are examples:

1. After-school bicycle races with an intermission devoted to a police officer discussing safe bicycle riding practices.
2. Initiations into the bicycle gang requiring the passing of a bicycle safety knowledge quiz.
3. A schoolwide auditorium program devoted to bicycling safety created and conducted by the bicycle gang.
4. A school newsletter emphasizing bicycling safety published by the gang.
5. A biking trip organized for a Saturday, requiring all bicyclers to pass a bicycle safety knowledge quiz before being permitted to participate.

Since bicycling has become so popular, high school and junior high school students will enjoy this activity greatly.

Safety Surveys

To understand where one should go, one should know where one has been. Similarly, if the safety-related behavior of students is to be affected in home and at school, they must investigate the present state of safety at those places. Once a picture of home and school safety behaviors has been uncovered, the next appropriate step would be to recommend improvements in this picture. The following two surveys can be employed to develop the safety picture of home and school. One word of caution: These questionnaires represent the ideal. The home and school should not be placed in a defensive position through the administration of these surveys. Before responding to the questionnaires, parents and school personnel should understand the nature of this investigation; i.e., to enable the students to make recommendations and *work with* parents and school personnel to improve upon the safety at these two places.

Is this true of our school?	Yes	Partly	No
1. The school administration takes a direct and personal interest in planning and carrying out a schoolwide safety education program.	—	—	—
2. Throughout the school program, the administration emphasizes the development of safety consciousness.	—	—	—
3. The principal facilitates and actively promotes the integration of safety instruction with all curriculum areas and co-curricular activities.	—	—	—
4. The school has a procedure whereby pupils, teachers, and custodians may submit suggestions regarding hazardous conditions and practices they observe in the school environment.	—	—	—

Yes **Partly** **No**

5. A qualified faculty member provides necessary leadership and guidance for including appropriate learning experiences in safety throughout all phases of the school program and at all levels.

6. Classroom teachers understand the importance of appropriate organization and supervision of pupil activities.

7. The school has a definite procedure to be followed in case of accident, and the plan is understood by classroom teachers, staff members, and students.

8. Pupils and classroom teachers, upon first entering school, and at the beginning of the year, are given full instructions on exit drills.

9. All pupils, classroom teachers, and staff members have a clear working knowledge of the exit drill directions and rules.

10. Teachers and students receive instruction and practice in how to meet such emergencies as blocked exits and blocked stairways during exit drills.

11. Classroom teachers and pupils evaluate each exit drill so that improvements may be made in procedures for evacuating the building.

12. All classroom teachers, custodians and other staff members have had instruction and practice in using different types of fire extinguishers.

13. A school person has been designated responsibility for directing the school civil defense program.

14. Appropriate civil defense emergency services such as fire, rescue, first aid, and engineering have been organized within the school.

15. Shelter area drills for the entire school are held frequently to prepare everyone for an emergency.

16. Each drill is evaluated to reveal weaknesses in planning, coordination, and communication.

17. Responsibilities of school personnel for safety and safety education are discussed regularly at faculty meetings.

18. All classroom teachers understand that safety education becomes effective when it is integrated naturally and logically with all curriculum areas and with all school activities.

19. Through in-service programs and other means, all

	Yes	Partly	No

teachers have an opportunity to learn what constitutes safe practices in a school program. — — —

20. Drills are held regularly in which riders, assisted by the school bus patrol, evacuate the bus by way of the emergency door. — — —

21. Pupils who ride school buses have an opportunity to take part in developing safety regulations for their own observance. — — —

22. Students and teachers are required to wear appropriate personal protective equipment such as safety goggles, aprons, and gloves during the more hazardous operations in special activity rooms. — — —

23. Safety education is a definite, important part of the educational program. — — —

24. The principal or another professional staff member serves as a leader to facilitate facultywide, schoolwide activities in safety education. — — —

25. Teachers of safety education are provided with adequate instructional materials. — — —

26. Safety education is included in continuous curriculum planning. — — —

27. All teachers are encouraged to:

   a) Attend classes in safety education conducted at colleges and universities. — — —

   b) Participate in in-service safety education programs of the school system. — — —

28. Classroom instruction in safety includes consideration of environmental hazards (school, home, highway, fire, recreational, and occupational) and provides opportunity for each pupil to develop a foundation for safe behavior patterns. — — —

29. The content of safety instruction is integrated wherever it fits naturally and logically with the subject matter in all curriculum areas and in all school activities. — — —

30. The following methods and devices are typical of those used in the program of safety instruction:

   a) Pupil discussions directly related to the safe and effective use of equipment and materials in various classes. — — —

   b) Motion pictures and filmstrips dealing with various aspects of safety. — — —

	Yes	Partly	No

c) Dramatizations of reading materials on safety.

d) Supplementary reading materials on safety.

e) Pictures and posters concerned with safety.

f) Student organizations, such as safety committees and student councils.

g) School patrols (building, bus, civil defense, exit drills, playground, and street traffic).

h) Talks to classes and assemblies by policemen, firemen, and other specialists.

31. Students demonstrate a feeling of responsibility for safe conditions and practices in and around the school.

32. The school has available and regularly uses safety materials which:

a) Motivate activities involving learning by doing.

b) Reflect currently accepted educational practice.

c) Relate naturally to program objectives.

d) Emphasize positive rather than negative aspects of safety education.

e) Are suited to students' maturity levels, needs, and interests.

f) Come from reliable sources.

g) Were developed by professional educators.

33. The school library has materials for both teachers and students on various phases of safety which meet the above criteria.

34. The school newspaper devotes special issues, or space in regular issues, to safety activities in the school program.

35. Textbooks used in the various curriculum areas include pertinent material in safety.

36. Accident statistics from the local area (city, county, or state) are studied as a part of the safety education program.

37. Posters made by students and also those obtained from outside sources are used to further safety instructions.

38. The local building and fire departments, or other reliable agencies, inspect the school building periodically in a continuing effort to reduce accident and fire hazards.

	Yes	Partly	No

39. The principal or a schoolwide safety committee has asked the following sources for safety materials:

   a) Office of local school system.   —   —   —

   b) State education department.   —   —   —

   c) Colleges and universities.   —   —   —

   d) Organizations interested in safety education.   —   —   —

   e) Business and industry groups.   —   —   —

    These checklists are designed to call special attention to safe living practices, techniques, and facilities that are frequently violated. Point out to the students that they should answer the questions honestly, and that the checklists will not be collected.

Home safety habits   Yes   No

1. Do you consciously look for hazards as you go about your daily work?   —   —

2. Do you use nonflammable cleaning fluids only for minor spot removal? Do you use them outside or in areas of good cross-ventilation?   —   —

3. Do you always disconnect portable electric appliances at the outlet when you've finished using them?   —   —

4. Do you dry your hands thoroughly before connecting or disconnecting electric equipment?   —   —

5. Are all bleaches, cleaning compounds, lye, and similar supplies kept locked and out of reach of children?   —   —

6. Do you observe the manufacturer's instructions when using appliances?   —   —

7. Do you apply floor wax in a thin coat and polish it thoroughly to reduce slipping hazards?   —   —

8. When lifting, do you bend your leg muscles and keep your chin in to avoid back injuries?   —   —

Home inspections   Yes   No

1. Do you have chimneys and heating equipment inspected regularly?   —   —

2. Are your basement and attic free of accumulations of rubbish, newspapers, and flammable materials?   —   —

3. Do you regularly clean the workshop, basement, and garage?   —   —

4. Are scatter rugs fastened down, laid on nonskid pads or treated with nonslip material? — —

5. Are all platforms, stair treads, and porch steps in good repair? — —

6. Is your yard free of broken glass, nail-studded boards, garden tools, and other litter? — —

7. Do you replace or repair worn floor coverings? — —

8. Are all flammable liquids stored in tight metal containers away from heat? — —

9. Do you repair or replace worn or frayed cords and plugs on lamps, appliances, motors, and tools? — —

10. Do you keep steps clear of clutter? — —

Home safety features   **Yes No**

1. Are handrails securely installed along the full length of all stairways? — —

2. For better visibility, are the top and bottom steps of outside stairs painted white or marked with luminous tape? — —

3. Are stairways and landings well lighted so the edge of each step is clearly visible? — —

4. Are electrical outlets well-placed and distributed, so that if you must use an extension cord you can avoid stretching it across work surfaces, sinks and traffic paths? — —

5. Are there enough electrical outlets, so that the use of extension cords can be avoided? — —

6. Are closets well-lighted? Do they have strong shelves and rods? — —

7. Are window screens and storm sashes securely fastened? — —

8. Is your roof covered with a fire-resistant material such as asphalt shingles? — —

9. Is your laundry equipment grounded through the use of three-prong outlets? — —

10. Do you have night-lights in bedrooms or halls? — —

11. Do all appliances have the Underwriters' Laboratories label? — —

12. Do you have a storage rack for sharp knives, scissors, and other utensils? — —

13. Is the medicine cabinet placed out of the reach of children? If not, do you keep it locked? — —

14. Do you have a sturdy step-ladder that is lightweight and easy to handle? — —

15. Do you have covered metal containers for storage of cleaning cloths that have absorbed oils, grease, or paint? — —
16. Do you have a first aid kit handy? Do you have an elementary knowledge of first aid procedure? — —

VALUING ACTIVITIES

Included below are but some examples of how values clarification may be applied to the study of physical health content.

Values Statements

Students can be asked to complete unfinished sentences which will manifest their values regarding physical health. The following stems of questions are suggested:

My body_____

Bathing_____

Flossing my teeth_____

Sneezing_____

Measles_____

An ill friend_____

Sleeping is_____

Amniocentesis_____

Circadian rhythms_____

Flu vaccine_____

Values Voting

The following questions can be posed by the teacher with the students voting yes or no on each. Discussion should be allowed to interrupt the voting at any time.

How many of you would have a heart transplant if that was needed to lengthen your life?

How many of you think that women live longer than men because of different life styles?

How many of you take vitamins daily?

How many of you get regular physical examinations?

How many of you would have a second child if your first child was born genetically ill?

How many of you stay away from other people when you have a cold?

How many of you brush and floss your teeth daily?

How many of you get enough sleep?

How many of you feel better in the morning than later in the day?

How many of you often feel tense?

Consistency Check[16]

The Consistency Check is an interesting way to consider the degree to which students behave consistently with their thoughts and/or feelings. Ask students to fill out this handout.

1. You have an important test to take but you wake up that morning with a 101° fever. Relative to attending school:

   What are you thinking you should do?_____

   _____

   How do you feel?_____

   _____

   What would you usually do?_____

   _____

   How consistent is your behavior with your thoughts and/or feelings?_____

   _____

Other leading statements which can be considered similarly are:

1. It's a Saturday and when you awaken you notice it is only 8 a.m. Regarding the choice of whether you go back to sleep or wake up.
2. You are contemplating flossing your teeth but you would rather watch television.
3. You are in a car with an adult who is smoking a cigarette.
4. One of your friends is making fun of someone who practices transcendental meditation twice daily.
5. A teacher is doing something that is unhealthy.
6. You have sickle-cell trait and want to marry someone who also has sickle-cell trait.
7. A classmate of yours is having an epileptic seizure.
8. A close friend is told by a physician that he or she has terminal cancer.

Values Continuum

For each of the questions below, ask students to place themselves on the continuum:

```
L_____|_____J
Always                                          Never
```

1. I brush my teeth daily.
2. I floss my teeth daily.
3. Physical health is more important than mental health.
4. Appearance is more important than health.
5. Schools are concerned with students' health.
6. My teacher is healthy.
7. It's as important to smell good as to be healthy.
8. I use a deodorant.
9. I use hair spray.
10. Epileptics who have seizures should be allowed to participate in school sports.
11. People with sickle-cell trait should be allowed to marry.
12. Married couples who have a history of mental retardation in either family should have children.
13. Children not inoculated against childhood diseases should be allowed to attend school.
14. I wash my hands before eating anything.
15. Candy machines should be allowed in school buildings.

Values Sheet

The purpose of this activity is to explore personal health behavior and to relate personal values to that behavior. Students are given a handout on which is presented a statement for their consideration. After the statement is read they are to answer the questions below it. Here is an example of a values sheet which concerns itself with physical health behavior:

Each of us has habits which can be considered healthy; and each of us has habits that are unhealthy. Considering your *physical* health: What three habits of yours can you think of that are unhealthy?

1. _____

2. _____

3. _____

Why do you do these things?

1. _____

2. _____

3. _____

What are the consequences of continuing these unhealthy behaviors?

1. _____

2. _____

3. _____

Filling In Blanks

Still another means of exploring the values behind unhealthy behaviors is to fill in blanks of sentences designed for this purpose. Once the value is identified, other more healthy behaviors may be substituted that will meet the same needs. An example of the standard sentences which can be used for this purpose is:

I (unhealthy behavior) because it (why you do it). The value underlying this behavior is (the value). A more healthy way of achieving this need would be (healthy behavior). I (will or will not) (the new behavior) by (date).

These completed sentences might appear as:

I smoke cigarettes because it makes me appear grown up. The value underlying this behavior is independence. A more healthy way of achieving this need would be earning money at a job after school. I will get a job by two weeks from today.

Students should be asked to keep a record of these completed sentences in a personal diary, and to note which timetables have been met and which have not. In this way, students will be required to assume responsibility for their own health-related behavior.

Giving Up

This activity can be used to achieve several health education objectives: It can help students to experience the difficulty one has in quitting smoking; it can help students appreciate the difficulty of living one's life with a handicap that prohibits particular behaviors (e.g., no contact sports for a child with a plastic heart valve insert); or it can be used to demonstrate the relative values of maintenance of physical health versus short-term gratification. When it is used for this latter purpose, students are asked to give up, for one week, something *important to them*. Some may choose not to watch television for a week, others to not eat snacks between meals that week, or still others to refrain from sports activities that week. Whatever is given up, however, must be valued by the student giving it up. At the conclusion of that week, the students are asked to consider the following:

1. How difficult was it giving up something you valued? Explain.
2. How did you feel the first time you were able to, once again, do the thing you gave up?
3. How did you feel when you did it?
4. Did you substitute anything during the week for the thing you gave up? If yes, what was it?
5. Do you value the thing you gave up more now than before you gave it up?
6. Are there some people who can never, for whatever reason, do the thing you gave up? (For instance, people who are blind can never watch television.)
7. How do you think they feel?
8. What could you do for such a person if you knew one?
9. What other conditions result in having to give things up?
10. Do people with such conditions find other things to value? Or do they find other activities to manifest their values?

The Patient

A game that will help students explore the consequences of uncontrolled communicable diseases and to examine the values involved in the decision-making process related to such diseases, involves them responding in small groups to the following handout:[17]

> You are a highly trained group called County Medical Helpers. Each of you has been specifically trained to administer first aid, recognize communicable diseases, and set up appointments for the doctor. Your primary responsibilities are to visit the residents of your county and identify those people who are in need of medical assistance.
>
> The people in your rural community are poor and uneducated.
>
> There is only one traveling doctor who visits once a week. He makes the final diagnosis and treatment. The day before his regular visit you are informed that the doctor will have only enough time to see five patients. You are to bring them to the church basement, which is used for the doctor's office. Your group has identified ten people who need medical assistance. Your job is to select the five who will see the doctor.
>
> 1. Mary, age 79, severe cold, chronic cough, possible pneumonia.

2. John, age 15, suspected tuberculosis.

3. Bobby, age 9, sudden fever, weakness, coughing, aching pain in back and extremities, possible influenza.

4. Susan, age 19, home from college, symptoms indicate polio or mononucleosis.

5. Sam, age 24, syphillis.

6. Linda, age 43, infectious hepatitis.

7. Mary, age 5, trachoma.

8. Virginia, age 7, smallpox.

9. Charles, age 54, cholera.

10. Butch, age 29, polio.

The following questions then give focus to a discussion of this activity:

1. Did all group members agree upon the five patients who were to see the doctor?

2. What considerations were given to your choices?

3. Which five did your group select and why?

4. What are the consequences, if any, for those patients not selected?

5. What might have been done to prevent these ten people from acquiring their disease?

CONCLUSION

Physical health can be investigated as a topic in and of itself. When this occurs, less traditional (and usually more exciting and interesting) topics can be studied along with the usual content of communicable diseases, safety, physical fitness, dental health, and physiology. However, even when the more traditional content areas are being studied, the student-centered activities in this chapter will make that study more interesting and result in greater learning than might otherwise have occurred.

REFERENCES

1. CRM Books, *Instructor's Guide to Life and Health* (New York: Random House, 1972), p. 87. Used by permission.

2. Lucien Brouha, "The Step Test: A Simple Method of Measuring Physical Fitness for Muscular Work in Young Men," *Research Quarterly* **14,** 1 (1943), p. 31.

3. J. Roswell Gallagher and Lucien Brouha, "A Simple Method of Testing the Physical Fitness of Boys," *Research Quarterly* **14,** 1 (1943), p. 23.

4. Edmund Jacobson, *Progressive Relaxation* (Chicago: University of Chicago Press, 1938).

5. Edmund Jacobson, *Teaching and Learning: New Methods for Old Arts* (Chicago: National Foundation for Progressive Relaxation, 1973).

6. J. H. Schultz and W. Luthe, *Autogenic Training: A Psychophysiological Approach to Psychotherapy* (New York: Grune & Stratton, 1959).

7. See: Robert Keith Wallace, Herbert Benson, and Archie F. Wilson, "A Wakeful Hypometabolic Physiologic State," *American Journal of Physiology*, Sept. 1971, p. 795; or Robert Keith Wallace and Herbert Benson, "The Physiology of Meditation," *Scientific American*, Feb. 1972, p. 84; or Robert Keith Wallace, "Physiological Effects of Transcendental Meditation," *Science* **167** (1970), pp. 1751–1754.

8. Herbert Benson, John F. Beary, and Mark P. Carol, "The Relaxation Response," *Psychiatry*, Feb. 1974, p. 37.

9. Readers interested in this subject should see: Julia Donnell, "Performance Decrement As a Function of Total Sleep Loss and Task Duration," *Perceptual and Motor Skills* **29** (1969), pp. 711–714; E. L. Hartman, *The Function of Sleep* (New Haven: Yale University Press, 1973); Yoshio Sarto, "Specification of Variation Patterns of Physiological and Performance Measurement in Sleep Loss," *Journal of Human Ergology* **1** (1972), pp. 207–216.

10. Raymond H. Schmitt, "Sleep: An Instructional Unit," unpublished paper, April 1976. Used by permission.

11. Donald B. Stone, Lawrence B. O'Reilly, and James D. Brown, *Elementary School Health Education: Ecological Perspectives* (Dubuque, Iowa: Wm. C. Brown, 1976), p. 366.

12. Ibid., p. 366.

13. Marvin Karlins and Lewis M. Andrews, *Biofeedback: Turning On the Power of Your Mind* (New York: Lippincott, 1972), p. 98.

14. From The National Safety Council, *Accident Facts,* 1974.

15. Ibid.

16. Adapted from Ronald Klein et al., *Search for Meaning* (Dayton, Ohio: Pflaum/Standard, 1974), p. 51.

17. From Ruth C. Engs, Eugene Barnes, and Molly Wantz, *Health Games Students Play* (Dubuque, Iowa: Kendall/Hunt, 1975), pp. 125–126. Used by permission.

Instructional Strategies for Emerging Health Concerns

10

T his chapter concerns itself with health content recently emerging as areas for study. The instructional activities included pertain to the aged and aging, death and dying, and ethical issues related to health.

THE AGED AND AGING

Certainly one aspect of health instruction must be the study of the aged and the aging process. Since the nature of life is the content of health education, to neglect the latter stages of life is to do a disservice to those engaged in the study—namely students. In addition, the study of the aged and the aging process will lead students to insights into their own lives through understanding of the aged's disappointments, joys, feelings about things left undone, accomplishments of which they are proud, etc. To help in this study the following activities are suggested.

Aged Visitors

One means of studying the aged is to talk with them. A most valuable, touching, and enjoyable experience is to invite to class, and spend a session or two with, several elderly people. The visitors can be residents of an old-age home, members of a golden-age club, or grandparents of students in the class. Questions and topics for discussion should be developed by the students prior to the visitors' arrivals and screened by a representative for the invited guests, so as to ensure that the aged can deal psychologically with the items proposed. For instance, questions pertaining to the imminence of death for the aged and questions related to feelings about dying might be very much out of place for some groups and perfectly acceptable to others.

The experience of such visits will serve both the students and the aged well. The class will develop a greater appreciation for life by viewing it from "the other end," and the aged will be brought closer to life by socializing with the young and contributing to their education.

Adoptions

As a follow-up to class sessions in which the aged visit—or as a separate activity altogether—students can "adopt" an aged person. This adoption, of course, is not of a legal or binding nature, but represents a commitment on the part of the student to visit with the elderly person, keep that person in touch with the world, invite the adopted one to his or her home for a visit, etc. Obviously, the advantages of this activity are similar to those delineated above with the added

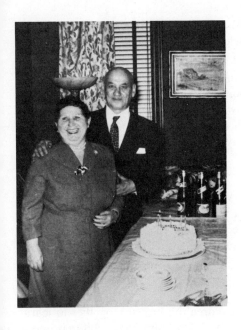

The aged should be seen by the young as enjoying life. Too often they are depicted as institutionalized, inactive, and just waiting for death. These people enjoyed themselves. I know. They were my grandparents.

opportunity for closer contact and a more intimate relationship than would otherwise be possible.

Phone Pal

Like having a pen pal with whom one exchanges letters on a periodic basis, students can choose phone pals. Phone pals should be residents of a nursing home or retirement home to whom students make telephone calls. Such calls should be devoted to establishing a relationship between the student and the aged, so as to improve upon the understanding of life for each. Several steps should be followed to set up the phone pal activity:

Step 1: The teacher should inquire of administrators of local nursing and retirement homes whether they would cooperate in such an activity.

Step 2: Those administrators approving of the project should identify certain of the aged as prospective phone pals.

Step 3: The prospective phone pals should be approached by the appropriate nursing home staff member to solicit their participation.

Step 4: Students should select a phone pal from a list of the aged willing to participate.

Step 5: Students should telephone the nursing home and arrange for personal visits with their phone pals.

Step 6: During the visit the phone pals should decide the time of day and days of the week (two or three) the telephone calls should be placed. During these visits telephone numbers of the phone pals should be exchanged.

Step 7: The activity is then conducted until such time as one or both of the callers decide it should be abandoned. The disengagement of pals should be conducted with the prior knowledge of the instructor so as to allow him or her some input into such a process. In this manner, a sense of rejection on the part of the elderly may best be avoided.

Visits To

Whereas elderly people can be asked to visit the class, the class can also visit the elderly. Such visits might consist of a walk, talk, or other informal activity. However, more planned activities can be arranged, such as the performing of skits, arts and crafts sessions, or the sharing of gifts made by students.

DEATH AND DYING

A classroom is a unique setting in which children are brought together to learn. It seems reasonable to assume that by the act of forming these children into a *group* for learning, something is planned which could not be offered to these children individually at their home. What better reason for gathering people together than to provide an environment conducive to their interacting? And what better topic to talk about than something which is interesting, perplexing, confusing, and upsetting; which has been suppressed and repressed all our lives? Such a topic is death.

Children contact death in many ways: through the death of pets; in stories and books, songs, and television programs; by the death of loved ones; and by dissection of animals in school. Therefore, to attempt to protect children from death by ignoring the topic is ludicrous. "Mental health, the mental health of us all, child and adult, is not the denial of tragedy but the frank acknowledgment of it. . . . Where can one turn in tragedy? But if tragedy can be admitted, we shall find our comfort in what we can mean to each other."[1]

Seldom are children, or adults, provided the opportunity to vent feelings about death. Parents don't initiate such discussions, and in fact shy away from answering childrens' questions about death. Cartoon programs on television depict death in a bizarre manner. "Heroes and villians alike are shot with rifles, crushed by gigantic boulders, blown to pieces by dynamite, bombarded with cannon balls, and pushed off cliffs, only to jump to their feet (after the laughter stops) to be killed again."[2] Even hospitals segregate their morgue from the eyes of the public and patients, isolate dying patients (even though some research findings indicate that dying patients are better able to cope with their status if in contact with others not in such a condition), and often prohibit staff from referring to ward-mates who have died.

With a realization that death is a subject not responded to anywhere in our society though "present in our mental functioning at all times,"[3] it seems appropriate for schools and, in particular, health educators, to organize activities which result in a study of death and dying, and which allow for the venting of feelings regarding one's own death. An important consideration, though, is the manner in which such activities are conducted. If the scientific method is employed in schools, the teacher who finds the child questioning the values of our society and religious teaching should not be surprised. "Children in our primary schools are making observations of the 'cycle of Nature,' including death and disintegration, and at the same time are being taught that Jesus 'ascended into heaven'."[4] In addition to the scientific inquiry into death and dying, the teacher should employ activities designed to elicit feeling about these topics. In conducting these activities, though, it is wise to remember that "well-meaning adults often shower them (children) with verbal reassurance, giving them no time to express their own thoughts."[5]

To conclude this introduction to activities related to death and dying, we should get rid of the attitude that "when I am, Death is not. . . . When death is, I am not. Therefore, we can never have anything to do with death?"[6] It is wise to remember "Socrates . . . died in good cheer and in control, unlike the agony of Jesus with his deep human cry of desertion and loneliness. Americans tend to behave as Socrates did. But there is more of what Jesus stands for lurking in our unconscious. . . ."[7] With the need for death education as just described, the following activities are recommended.

Run For Your Life

A television series entitled "Run For Your Life" had as its theme the predicted near death of its star character. This character was told at the series outset that he had a terminal illness and had a year or two of life remaining. He decided to cram a lifetime of adventure into his two remaining years, and the show followed its star about the world as he sped around tracks with his racing car, made deep sea dives and sky dives, and fell repeatedly in love.

Using a similar theme, students can be asked to role-play being placed in a like position: being told that they are terminally ill. Once placed in that role, they are asked to describe how they would spend their time. An analysis of these descriptions might involve the following queries:

1. At what places did you choose to spend your time? Why there?
2. With whom did you choose to spend your time? Why?
3. Whom did you exclude from spending time with that you usually do? Why?
4. What did you spend your time doing? Why? Do you *presently* spend your time in this way?
5. What can be concluded from the answers to the questions appearing above?

The results of this activity will evidence two factors in particular: (1) students (people) differ in their values, as indicated by the priorities they set for their most precious commodity—i.e., time—and (2) some students tend to spend a significant amount of their time doing the things they feel are important, at places enjoyable to them, with people with whom they like to spend time, whereas others do not. With this activity, the threat of death can be used as a positive force to make more sense out of life.

Death Completions

To allow students the opportunity to show their feelings about death, they can be asked to complete the following sentences which will then be discussed in small groups:

1. Death is_____
2. I would like to die at_____
3. I don't want to live past_____
4. I would like to have at my bedside when I die_____
5. When I die, I will be proud that when I was living I_____
6. My greatest fear about death is_____
7. When I die, I'll be glad that when I was living I didn't_____
8. If I were to die today, my biggest regret would be_____
9. When I die, I will be glad to get away from_____
10. When I die, I want people to say_____

Possessions

It has often been said that one's views of death determine how one lives. Those believing in life after death, for instance, can be expected to live in such a way as to improve their likelihood of a good afterlife. Those not believing in life after death might behave hedonistically so as to get pleasure out of life now, rather than postpone a great deal of pleasure for a later existence. One aspect of death sometimes neglected by teachers of health education relates to life's possessions. Possessions, and what one decides to do with these upon one's death, can reveal much about one's life. To investigate this relationship ask the class to respond to the following questions:

1. Which ten things that you own do you most cherish?
2. Why are these so dear to you?
3. Which of these do you expect to own twenty years from now?
4. Which of these have you already owned for several (two) years?

5. Which *three* of the ten possessions you cited before are most cherished by you? Why?
6. What do you want to happen to these ten possessions when you die?

This activity will require students to reevaluate the importance of things they own and how they behave regarding these items. For example, do they prohibit brothers or sisters from playing their records, records which are of value for such short duration? Do they treat others' possessions casually, while expecting their possessions to be handled with care? Are they more concerned with things than with people? The answers to these questions and others can be used by students to draw conclusions about how they behave, and how they would like to behave—which can then be integrated into their patterns of living.

Last Will

As a follow-up to the previous exercise, students should be asked to list as many of their possessions as come to mind. After this list is complete, students should write a last will and testament, in which they designate what is to be done with their possessions. The same objectives will be achieved as in the Possessions exercise.

Interruption

One of the concerns often expressed about death is that it interrupts the achieving of one's goals for life—that is, people feel that they will die with goals left unaccomplished. These goals can vary from person to person, but the feeling of interruption by death is fairly common. An activity to help students recognize this feeling in themselves and to organize their lives in ways in which this feeling is taken into account is described below.

Ask students to complete a chart which requires them to establish goals for each decade of their lives as follows:

Decade	Goal
0–10	
11–20	
21–30	
31–40	
41–50	
51–60	
61–70	
71–80	

When the chart is completed, the teacher asks the following:

1. Rank these goals in order of importance.

2. Cross out the goals already achieved.

3. If you were to die ten years from now, which goals would not have been accomplished?

4. Of these *un*accomplished goals if you died ten years from now, how many are in the top four?

5. Can these goals be reorganized so that those more important to you (as indicated by your rankings) can be achieved earlier in your life? If so, which?

6. Are there goals you would like to add? If so, where would you place them in terms of importance? Where would you place them in terms of decades of your life?

Tell Someone

A simple exercise, but one with a great deal of significance, requires students to conduct introspection. Many people, upon the death of a loved one, will bemoan their not having said to that loved one, "I love you dearly." This activity requires students to list the most important people in their lives. Next, the class is asked to place beside the names of those dear to them one thing they could tell these people which would enhance their lives upon the students' deaths. Lastly, the teacher challenges the students to actually approach these loved ones and say to them what they have written. Whether or not this latter phase of the activity is attempted is, of course, decided by the students. However, the thought has been planted, and the improvement of their relationships with those important to them has been made more possible. Again, as with the other exercises in this section, this exercise relates to the improvement of life and life relationships through the acceptance of the inevitability of death.

ETHICAL ISSUES

With the advance of science and the increasing sophistication of technology, new health-related considerations have presented themselves. Such considerations are:

1. When is a person dead? When is it proper to use his or her organs for transplant?

2. Does each person have the right to a timely death, as comfortable as possible? For how long should life sustaining machines be employed to maintain the life of a hopelessly ill patient?

3. Should medical researchers be permitted to experiment on live fetuses resulting from abortions?

4. Is the use of prison personnel for medical experimentation ethical? Should prisoners be tempted to risk their lives in such experiments through promises of a shorter internment?

5. When does life begin? At conception, birth, or sometime between the two? Does a fetus have rights? Are abortions ethical?

6. Is the fee-for-service health care system ethical? Does such a system discriminate against the poor? Do health maintenance organizations provide a more responsive system of health care?

7. When medical researchers are experimenting upon people, they are required to obtain informed consent. What constitutes informed consent? For incompetents, can parents, guardians or others give such consent? How much of the experiment must be understood by the consenter?

These issues and others have no easy answers. The medical community alone must not be expected to respond to such concerns without input from the citizenry. However, to provide necessary input for making decisions relative to these issues requires an understanding of them, and the implications associated with alternative responses for their solution. Since education in schools professes to prepare the young for their roles as citizens, and since today's youth will be expected to make tomorrow's decisions, it seems necessary to discuss ethical issues related to health in health education classes. To wait until an issue becomes a severe problem, rather than respond to issues at their outset, represents a head-in-the-sand approach not advocated here. Health education itself is preventive in nature, and so should be our responses to societal concerns.

Activities follow to help teachers present ethical concerns to students; but perhaps the best way to emphasize the importance of prevention and early intervention as described above is with the following poem:[8]

> Twas a dangerous cliff, as they freely confessed,
> Though to walk near its crest was so pleasant;
> But over its terrible edge there had slipped
> A duke, and full many a peasant.
> The people said something would have to be done,
> But their projects did not at all tally.
> Some said, "Put a fence 'round the edge of the cliff";
> Some, "An ambulance down in the valley."
> The lament of the crowd was profound and was loud,
> As their hearts overflowed with their pity;
> But the cry for the ambulance carried the day
> As it spread through the neighboring city,
> A collection was made to accumulate aid,
> And the dwellers in highway and alley
> Gave dollars or cents—not to finish a fence—
> But an ambulance down in the valley.
> The story looks queer as we've written it here,
> But things oft occur that are stranger,
> More humane, we assert, than to succor the hurt,
> Is the plan of removing the danger.
> The best possible course is to safeguard the source;

Attend to things rationally.
Yes, build up the fence, and let us dispense
With the ambulance down in the valley."

Euthanasia

To force students to face the issue of when not to sustain life,[9] present to them a handout on which appears the following critical incident:[10]

> Ken and Cheryl Bater had been married just four months when they found out for sure that she was pregnant. Ken picked her up at the doctor's office that afternoon, and before the dinner dishes were washed they had chosen two names—Claudia for a girl, Todd if it turned out to be a boy. Then, the teenage newlyweds made long-term plans as they happily faced the responsibilities of parenthood. They opened their first savings account. Ken cut his beer budget in half. Cheryl began preparing the house. Their lives were now wrapped up in anticipation of that day in mid-November when the baby would arrive.

> Everything went well until one October afternoon when Ken's foreman called him off the assembly line to the phone. "Just listen," Cheryl ordered, her voice edged with tears. "I'm going to the hospital in a taxi. I think the baby might be coming early." No, she couldn't be positive. "But Ken, you've got to meet me there," she said. "And hurry, please."

> Todd was born 90 minutes later—six weeks premature—weighing barely four pounds. He was weak, and it was immediately obvious that he had serious respiratory problems. The doctor could not get him to breathe on his own.

> A few years ago Todd would have died at birth. But now, even at the modest-sized, midwestern hospital where the drama of Cheryl and Ken and Todd unfolded, new techniques and equipment have dramatically reversed the odds of survival for babies with acute problems.

> Todd was rushed from the delivery room to the intensive-care nursery and placed in an incubator with an infant respirator attached. This machine actually breathes for the baby until, hopefully, his own lungs can take over the job.

> "Don't worry, we'll pull the little fella through," John Filipelli, M.D., assured Ken and Cheryl. But what the pediatrician did not tell them was that there was a significant chance that Todd had suffered lasting brain damage as a result of the oxygen deficiency he experienced just after birth.

> In a few days, Cheryl went home. But Todd remained in the hospital, still under intensive care, on and off the respirator. One week stretched to two and then four. Still, the infant did not fully respond. His weight hovered around five pounds. Each new breathing crisis increased the likelihood that his brain would sustain permanent damage from the lack of oxygen.

> Nurses on the 3 P.M. to 11 P.M. shift, the hours when Ken and Cheryl visited, were becoming increasingly concerned, both for the young parents whom they watched sadly gaze at their struggling son, and for the baby himself.

> "Poor kids," a floor nurse said after the couple had left one day in November. "I wonder how much they know—I bet if they knew that they might wind up

with just half a child, they wouldn't want us to keep putting him back on the respirator every time he has a failure."

"If it were up to me," said the nurse checking the gauges, "the next time we take him off, if he can't make it on his own, I would just let him go."

What would you do?

The teacher should then form small groups to discuss what each student's reaction would be in the case described. After twenty minutes of such discussion, the following handout, which completes the story, should be distributed:[11]

The medical staff has been calling on Frank Reidy for eight years. He took the job as the first staff chaplain at the hospital only after being assured by the administration that he was to be "an ethical consultant to the medical staff as well as performing the usual handholding service and dispensing the death notices." In fact, he still has a copy of the letter with these words underlined. An ordained Lutheran minister, Chaplain Reidy has earned a reputation for asking the kind of direct questions that doctors and hospital administrators often find painful. (The chaplain, the doctor, and the Baters are all real people, and the events described here really happened in a regional hospital somewhere in the Midwest. Their names have been changed to protect their privacy and legal rights.)

Picking up the telephone in his office near the waiting room, Frank Reidy immediately recognized the voice of the nurse on the other end. "You sound upset, Barbara. What's up? . . . Of course, I'll be up in a minute. By the way, who's the doctor? . . . Oh sure, I know John Filipelli. Okay, well I'm on my way."

As the chaplain rounded the last corner on his way toward the nurseries, he was deep in thought. "Frank? . . . Is that you?" The voice that interrupted him from behind belonged to John Filipelli. They talked about the Bater's baby.

"Before you make any decision about the baby, I think you have to be sure that you have eliminated any prejudices you have," Chaplain Reidy was telling Dr. Filipelli. "Once you are sure that you have done all you can, you should try to get into it from the parents' point of view—and even from the baby's. First, though: Are you sure that you haven't kept the child alive this long out of some sense of guilt on your part?"

"No, no. There's nothing like that," the pediatrician answered quickly. Then a pause. "At least nothing about the baby. At the start though, when I first met the parents, I might have gone a little too strong in assuring them that the kid would be okay. I feel badly about that now, sure. But I don't think 'guilty' is the word. Still, now that I stop to really think about it, I guess something like that *could* have influenced me to push just a little harder to keep the baby alive— against better judgment. Another thing, too, is that the longer the baby is up there the bigger the bill gets. I suppose that insurance will pay most of it, but it must be over $5,000 by now. I guess what I am saying is that it becomes even harder to pull the plug after we all have put so much into it. Yet the longer I keep putting him on the respirator, the less the chances are that they will have an intact baby in the end. The chances of brain damage are already awfully high, to say nothing of his physical problems which haven't stabilized."

The doctor was almost talking to himself now. His head bent, staring into the cold, stagnant cup of coffee in front of him, his thoughts trailed into silence. Suddenly he looked up, remembering where he was and relieved to see that he and the chaplain were still alone in the snack bar. No strangers were close enough to have overheard his self-doubt.

"How much do you know about the parents?" Reidy asked. "Have you talked to them honestly about all this?"

"Oh come off it, Frank," the doctor exploded. "They're kids themselves. You can't ask them to make this kind of decision. What do you want me to do—walk up to them and say, 'Okay, what do we do: kill your child or give him back to you as a vegetable?' Heck, every time they go into the nursery, they look scared stiff," the doctor rebutted.

"Maybe they wouldn't be so scared if they knew what was going on, if you hadn't tried to protect them from the start. Are you sure that part of the problem isn't that you are copping out of facing them? Don't forget: It's *their* child, and they are the ones who are getting up to their necks in debt.

"By the way, do you actually know how important money is to them?" The minister's questions were jolting.

"Maybe they have more money than you do. And one other thing that's probably important: Is there any reason why the mother can't carry another child? If there is, you know they are going to try everything to save this one, no matter how badly damaged it is."

The doctor stood and slowly walked across the room to a window overlooking a dreary parking lot. For nearly a full minute he watched the patterns of raindrops splashing below. "Look, Frank," he finally said. "You've been a big help. You always are. I need a few minutes to sort some of this out alone. Then I want to call her doctor and see if he can give me answers to some of those questions. Why don't you tell the nurses that we talked and ask them to page me when the parents come in this afternoon. Then I may want you to talk to them after I have seen them. Okay?"

"If you need me I'll be in my office or up on the dialysis unit. There's a tough one up there today, too," the chaplain said. "Do you know what you are going to tell the parents?"

"I'm going to tell them that I think we should switch the respirator from 'control' to 'assist' if Todd has to go back on it again. The machine will help him keep himself alive, but it won't force him to breathe if he wants to stop. At least that's what I think we should do," Dr. Filipelli said.

After Ken and Cheryl Bater heard John Filipelli's recommendation, they indeed wanted to talk to Frank Reidy. The chaplain assured them that their decision to follow the doctor's suggestion was morally sound and that they had done all they could. They waited at the hospital through the next several hours—long enough to again meet with Frank Reidy when he told them that Todd was dead.

Eyes were moist inside and outside the intensive-care nursery that afternoon as everyone worked through another of those hard decisions—the kind that have called for bioethics to come into being in medical centers everywhere.

Abortion Debate

Relative to controversial topics such as abortion, students should be reminded to consult their clergy and parents before deciding on the appropriateness of such action. However, an objective investigation can be conducted in class to analyze the arguments for and against such practice. One of the best ways to conduct such an investigation employs the debate technique.[12] Three students should argue for legalization of abortion and three against it. It seems to this author that the teacher should make sure that at least the following points are made during such a debate:

1. A hospital abortion is safer than a routine tonsillectomy.[13]
2. "Since 1869 some members of the Roman Catholic hierarchy have argued that the fetus is, from conception, a human being in the full sense of the term and that abortion is murder.

   Substantial non-Catholic theological opinion disagrees and, in fact, increasing numbers of Roman Catholic laymen do not feel that abortion is murder. They regard the fetus as a *potential* human being, whose interests are secondary to those of its mother."[14]
3. "Some people believe that abortion-on-demand gives to one person (the mother) the legal right to kill another (the baby) in order to solve the first person's social problem."[15]
4. An evaluation of New York State's 1970 abortion law allowing abortion-on-demand has indicated:[16]

   a) Fewer women are dying during pregnancy and childbirth.
   b) There has been a decline in hospital admissions for "botched" criminal abortions and self-abortion attempts.
   c) Fewer infants are dying in the first month and first year of life.
   d) In New York City, out-of-wedlock births have declined for the first time.

Living Will

The Living Will is a contract between a dying person on the one hand, and his or her loved ones and physicians on the other. This Will requests that no heroic life-sustaining attempts be made to endlessly prolong one's life, but rather that one be allowed to die with dignity and in peace when the time comes. The development of a Living Will is a procedure in which students can be asked to participate. As a result of this experience, students will have developed greater insight into the question of when one should be let die. The right-to-life and right-to-die arguments will inevitably enter into a discussion accompanying the development of the Living Will. Such questions as the following should be considered:

1. How expensive is it to use life-sustaining technology to prolong the life of a hopelessly ill patient? Who pays for these procedures?
2. Who should determine when to "pull the plug?"
3. Is such a contract legally binding? (The answer is that it is not)
4. Does a person have the right to die if he or she so chooses? If yes, then should suicide be permitted?

Still Other Ethics Activities

Activities described elsewhere in this book can also be adapted to the study of ethical issues related to health. The reader is directed to "Who Should Survive" and "Value Judgment" in Chapter 3 and "The Patient" in Chapter 9 for examples of such learning experiences.

VALUING ACTIVITIES APPLIED TO EMERGING HEALTH CONCERNS

Emerging health concerns such as health ethics, death and dying, and the aged and the aging process lend themselves very well to valuing activities. By definition, emerging health topics are new or have been given recent emphasis. Because of this newness, very few right or wrong answers can be provided students studying issues related to these topics. Consequently, an exploration of values underlying proposed alternative solutions to these issues seems appropriate. The activities to follow are designed for this purpose.

Values Ranking

The following groups of terms can be rank ordered and the rankings discussed in small groups:

1. Old	1. Family	1. Dying
2. Young	2. Independence	2. Dead
3. Middle aged	3. Friends	3. Pain

1. Abortion anytime mother decides to
2. Abortion with physician's approval only
3. Abortion never

If you were old and ill which would you prefer?
1. Living in a nursing home
2. Living in a hospital
3. Living with a relative

If you were dying, which would you prefer?
1. Letting nature take its own course

2. Letting physicians keep you alive by any means
3. Letting a close relative decide when physicians should "pull the plug"

When you die which would you prefer?
1. Burial
2. Cremation
3. Body donated to science

If you were to donate one of your organs, upon death, to another, which organ would it be?
1. Heart
2. Eyes
3. Kidneys

Survival

The following game will require students to discuss ethical issues without ever having to identify them as such. Students should be divided into small groups of from four to six members. One group will imagine that they are *physicians,* another that they are *politicians,* another that they are *teachers,* another that they are *clergymen,* and the last that they are *teenagers.* Each group will receive these instructions:

> It is anticipated that a nuclear holocaust is imminent. Many deaths will occur, but luckily some bomb shelters have been equipped to provide safety for a select few. Since only 100 people can live in these shelters, all but these 100 will die. It is your group's task to establish criteria for selecting which 100 people will be allowed to inhabit the bomb shelters.
> *Don't forget the role you are playing.*

After each group has determined the criteria they would use, have these listed on the chalkboard. Next, have a member of each group present the reasoning their group used in establishing these criteria. After all such presentations, drop the role playing and have the total class review each of the criteria on the board and decide whether or not they should keep it. At the conclusion of this exercise, the following questions can be used to bring ethical issues into greater focus:

1. Who has the right to determine who shall live and who shall die?
2. When other than a nuclear bombing might such a decision be necessary?
3. In each of these situations, who should make the decision?
4. What should be considered in making each of these decisions?
5. How should this country be preparing *now* for dealing with such ethical issues in the future?

Values Grid

The values grid technique described in Chapter 3 can also be employed to help students organize decisions related to ethical issues. The objective is similar to that of the survival activity just described. The items to be placed in the values grid can be viewed as occupations which are—or are not—important for a country to maintain. When the exercise is completed, the reasons for the placements within the grid should be discussed.

The values grid handout given to each student should appear as follows:

Assume that a nuclear holocaust about to occur will result in many deaths, but that this country has provided for bomb shelters to allow 100 people to live In the grid below, place the four occupations you feel are *very important* for the survivors to have, the four that are *important,* the four *somewhat important,* and the four *least important* in the columns under these headings.

	Very Important	Important	Somewhat Important	Least Important
1.				
2.				
3.				
4.				

Occupations

1. physicians	5. nurse	9. policeman	13. genetic counselor
2. teacher	6. clergyman	10. fireman	14. school child
3. engineer	7. mother	11. administrator	15. retiree
4. politician	8. father	12. dentist	16. physicist

Values Listings

This exercise asks students to list the 15 people with whom they most like to spend time. Once this list is complete, the following directions should be given:

1. Place an "O" next to anyone older than 50.
2. Place a "Y" next to anyone younger than 10.
3. Place a "D" next to the five people most likely to die first.
4. Place a "T" next to the five people you would most trust in a life-and-death situation.

5. Think of your three most valuable material possessions. Place a "G" next to the three people to whom you would give one of these possessions if you were to die today.

6. If you were told you were dying and could only say goodbye to five of the people on your list, who would they be? Place the letter "M" next to these people.

The following questions will afford the students participating in this exercise the opportunity for introspection not often provided in school settings:

1. After following the instructions above, did you think of people who weren't on your list but you would now like to include? Who are they? Why did you originally leave them off?

2. Do you enjoy spending time with younger people, people your own age, or those older? Why?

3. Relative to the people most likely to die first:

   a) Are they the oldest on your list?

   b) Do you now want to spend more time with them?

   c) What do you want to do with them before they die?

   d) Do you think they would guess that you would include them on such a list? Should you tell them you did?

4. If you were dying in a hospital would you want any of the five people you designated as the ones you most trust to decide when to "pull the plug?" Or is there someone else you would rather assign that responsibility?

5. How would you feel giving one of your most valued possessions to the people you designated with a "G" *now* rather than when you are dying? Would the meaning behind the gift be more valuable to you than the possession itself?

6. What have you learned from having participated in this exercise?

Values Behaving

To confront students with the inconsistency between their professed values and their behavior relative to emerging health concerns, they should complete the following handouts:

A. Briefly describe what you believe to be the typical day of a senior citizen resident of a nursing home: _____

_____

_____

_____

_____

Identify three things about this typical day that you would not like were you this senior citizen.

1. _____

2. _____

3. _____

What could you do for such a resident to help make one of these three things less troublesome? _____

_____

Are you going to do it?____When? _____

B. Do you believe legislation should allow for abortions or do you believe legislation should disallow abortions? Check one:____allow____disallow

Which branch or branches of your State government would be responsible for such legislation? _____

_____

Have you communicated your opinions to your elected representative to this branch of government? Check one:____yes____no

Are you going to?____When? _____

C. If you were to die right now, is there something you would regret never having done?____If so, what is it? _____

_____

Is there something you would regret not having told someone? What? Who?

_____

_____

Are you going to do that thing soon?____When? _____

Are you going to tell that person?____When? _____

Values Continuum

Health ethics, sometimes termed medical ethics or bioethics, have been related to such topics as the right to die, the right to live, abortion, informed consent, human experimentation, etc. Not enough thought has been given to the ethical implications of determining for others how they should behave. For example, is it ethical to decide that students should not engage in premarital sexual intercourse and then *program* them through learning experiences to behave accordingly?[17] Which behaviors are appropriate to *pre*scribe for people and which are not? The following handout, once completed, is a good discussion starter for this issue:

Where would you place the numbered items on the continuum below? Write the number at the appropriate place.

Should be a matter of choice	Depends on one's age	Should be talked into or out of

1. Smoking cigarettes
2. Using marijuana
3. Drinking alcohol
4. Attending church or synagogue
5. Being kind
6. Having a will and testament
7. Remaining a virgin
8. Eating a balanced meal
9. Brushing and flossing teeth
10. Crossing at corners
11. Petting
12. Having a Living Will
13. Having an abortion
14. Accepting euthanasia
15. Caring at home for an invalid parent
16. Accepting welfare payments
17. Applying for food stamps
18. Using paper that can be recycled
19. Being open and honest
20. Maintaining proper weight for one's height

Values Statements

As stated earlier, unfinished sentences can be used to explore values. The following sentence stems can be employed to consider values related to emerging health concerns:

1. Death_____
2. Dying_____
3. Living_____
4. Free choice_____

5. The aged_____

6. The aging process_____

7. Nursing homes_____

8. Euthanasia_____

9. I want to die when_____

10. Abortion is_____

11. When I die I'll miss_____

12. Ethics means_____

13. Sex for the aged_____

14. Social Security payments_____

15. The "plug" should be pulled when_____

CONCLUSION

The purpose of this chapter has been twofold: first, to present instructional strategies for health concerns of recent emphasis (the aged and aging, death and dying, and health ethics); and second, to illustrate how new health education topics can easily be adapted to the student-centered approach to health instruction. Regardless of the content being considered, a more interesting, exciting, and meaningful approach to that content is to actively involve the learner. This chapter has demonstrated that this involvement is possible when it is consciously sought.

REFERENCES

1. Earl Grollman, *Explaining Death to Children* (Boston: Beacon Press, 1967) p. ix.
2. Richard Dumont and Dennis Foss, *The American View of Death: Acceptance or Denial?* (Cambridge, Mass.: Schenkman, 1972), p. 35.
3. Ibid., p. 19.
4. Marjorie Mitchell, *The Child's Attitude to Death* (Suffolk, England: Pemberton, 1966), p. 27.
5. Grollman, *Explaining Death to Children*, p. 163.
6. Dumont and Foss, *The American View of Death*, p. 104.
7. Ibid.
8. From *Healthways* **12,** 3 (1957). Used by permission.
9. Euthanasia does not mean, in this context, the taking of life, but rather the cessation of heroic life sustaining efforts such as the use of technology common in today's hospital.

10. Dale Wittner, "Life or Death," *Today's Health,* published by the American Medical Association, March 1974, p. 48. Used by permission.

11. Ibid., p. 49.

12. For a more exact description of how to organize a debate see Chapter 4.

13. Association for the Study of Abortion, *Abortion and Health* (pamphlet), undated.

14. Ibid.

15. Hiltz Publishing Co., *Did You Know* (pamphlet), undated.

16. National Association for Repeal of Abortion Laws, *50 Physicians Evaluate Legal Abortion in New York* (pamphlet), undated.

17. For an elaboration of this question the reader is referred to Chapter 1 of this book.

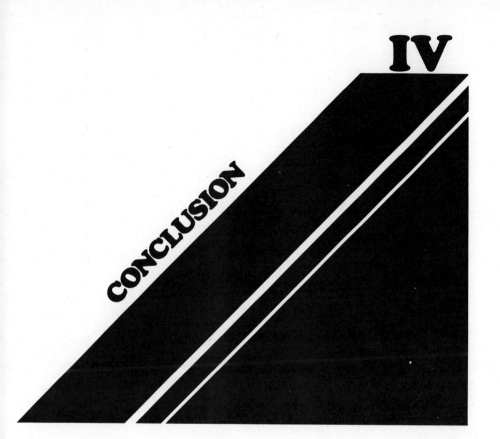

CONCLUSION

IV

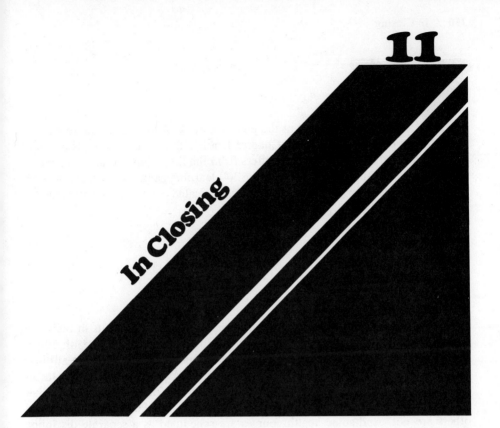

In Closing

11

What can be said at the end of a book of this sort? The reader can be reminded of the description in Chapter 1 of health instruction as it is presently constituted (and which admittedly suffers from the limitations of all such generalizations). The reason for presenting over 200 learning games and experiences can be reiterated. Or the hope for the future, indicated by the publication of this book, can be applauded.

Sounds good!

Let's try it all.

HEALTH EDUCATION NOW

Though many health education programs presently involve students in their own learning, many do not. The facilities and equipment provided to health educators are often substandard; the curriculum not sequential K–12; and the attitudes of parents, students, and fellow teachers not conducive to meaningful health instruction. Some health courses are required, others are not. Some health courses are assigned academic credit, others are not. Some health educators are certified, others are not. And some health courses are scheduled as a separate discipline, others are not.[1] In fact many health education programs:

1. Meet on rainy days or when the gymnasium is not being used for physical education.
2. Are not assigned one particular classroom so as to be able to store films, charts, cassettes, etc., but rather must transport these instructional materials from classroom to classroom.
3. Are bombarded with parental criticism relative to controversial content areas.
4. Are not seen as educationally valuable by fellow academicians.
5. Are viewed as bothersome and boring by students.
6. Are conducted by other than health educators.[2]

That there are some excellent health educators and health education programs attests to the potential, as yet not sufficiently tapped, of the discipline. These model programs tend to have several factors in common:

1. They are comprised of certified, qualified, and concerned health instructors.
2. They provide for instruction to occur outside, as well as inside, school walls.
3. They involve students significantly in the learning process.[3]

LEARNING EXPERIENCES IN THIS BOOK

The first of the three characteristics just mentioned as common to meaningful health education programs—that they are comprised of excellent health educators—is beyond the immediate influence of this author. However, the other two factors, learning outside school boundaries and significant involvement of students, have been the concerns of Chapters 2 through 10. In these chapters, over 200 learning activities have been described. Each of these activities seeks to actively involve students in their own learning by requiring them to uncover information, draw inferences, identify feelings, or discover insights by *their own* actions. The role of the teacher, then, is transposed from one of *being active* (lecturing) to one of *helping others be meaningfully active* (process leader, facilitator of learning, or whatever name suits the fancy of those who create pedagogical titles). Many of the activities described require the participation of people not associated with the school (e.g., the aged and aging section, Chapter 10), or require an environment other than the school for the activity to be conducted (e.g., home safety surveys, Chapter 9).

It should be noted, though, that while the activities included in this book are interesting and motivating for students, this is not justification alone for incorporating them into the reader's health education curriculum. The additional, and perhaps even more important, consideration is that they contribute to the achievement of objectives in health education. Cognizant of this concern, the author has related each learning experience to the health education objective that experience is designed to achieve. The reader should have clear in his or her own mind the reason for choosing a learning experience. Too often in the past, such games have been played in the classroom without the instructor being able to justify, educationally, their use.

THE HOPE FOR THE FUTURE

Several years back, a book of this sort would not have been able to be published. Health instruction, and education in general, was not considered to be fun. That is, learning was serious business consisting of hard work and extreme sacrifice. The fact that the reader is now holding this book in his or her hands attests to the direction in which all of education is moving—health education right along with the rest. The movement, entitled humanistic education, is toward the participation of students in a learning process whose objectives relate to the students knowing themselves, others, and their environments better than has routinely been the case. This author's hope is that, in some way, this book contributes to that movement.

However, the hope for the future, whose seeds are planted in today's humanistic education trends, lies further down the road of student involvement. Someday, schools will truly be service organizations whose doors will be open to those who have identified what they want to learn, have some idea as to how they want this learning to be conducted, and will recognize that they have achieved their objectives when, in fact, they have. Health educators, then, will be available to students to help them achieve *their* objectives in an interesting and educationally sound environment. Particular behaviors will not be predetermined as healthy, with students programmed to behave accordingly; rather, students will investigate the values systems they are and, with knowledge of themselves and health content, within societal limitations, determine for themselves what is healthy *for them*. If such an educational system seems difficult to imagine, think of those traditional educators to whom humanistic education was first proposed.

GETTING THERE

The teacher who wants to adopt a humanistic educational stance is advised to become familiar with the writings in this area. Too many wet their bodies in humanistic education before they see the need for swimming. One should understand the theory behind this type of education so as to be articulate in explaining that theory to parents, administrators, students, and colleagues. The reading list appearing in the appendix of this book should be helpful in this regard.

Next, a teacher might want to consider trying one or two of the activities in this book prior to "humanizing" totally. Different teacher and student personality mixes might necessitate local adaptations of the activities herein proposed. An initial, slow introductory phasing in of these activities and this approach to health instruction is therefore recommended.

In addition, teachers should not be afraid of consulting with colleagues who have employed more humanistic forms of education. Trial and error is only necessary where others have not tried before. Profit from the mistakes of the pioneers; don't repeat their mistakes. Students might also be able to provide feedback to the teacher so as to improve the attempt at a more humanistic mode of education.

Lastly, colleges often offer courses in humanistic education in which teachers could enroll. The teacher desiring to become more proficient in this educational approach should consult local colleges relative to such courses. Another such experience might be offered as in-service education by local school districts. Often experts in values clarification and/or humanistic education are brought to town by school districts with the goal of introducing such approaches to education to their teachers. Local newspapers usually announce such visits, so that paying attention to newspapers is a good means of becoming aware of the existence of visits by experts in valuing and humanistic education.

TO THE READER

It would be remiss of the author to conclude such a book without a personal (human, if you will) comment to the reader. Writing this book has been fun, hopefully profitable, and personally and professionally rewarding. However, only the reader can make the time spent on this project worthwhile. Only the employment of the activities included in this book, and the manifestation of concern for the students the author has attempted to convey, will make the time spent (the author's in writing and the reader's in reading) a useful, rather than wasteful, enterprise. As a football coach might say: The ball's in your hands—run with it.

Lastly, use the book in good health.

REFERENCES

1. See Chapter 1 for a more detailed discussion and justification of these statements.
2. Michigan Department of Education, *Patterns and Features of School Health Education in Michigan Public Schools* (Michigan: Department of Education, 1969), pp. 7–8.
3. To choose objectives, content, learning experiences, and means of evaluation; all to varying degrees.

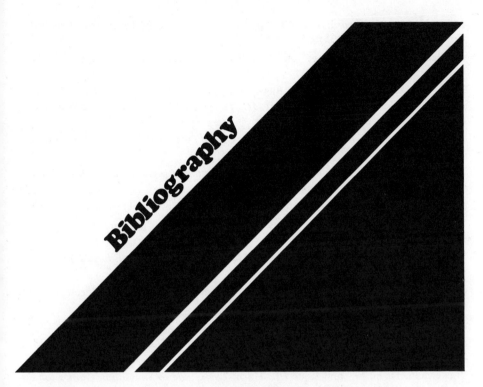

A. GENERAL GAMING-TYPE INSTRUCTIONAL STRATEGIES

The sources cited in this section of the bibliography include instructional activities which, though not specific to health education, can be adapted to that subject area. Consistent with the focus of this book, these activities are designed to require the active participation of the learner.

Abt, Clark C., *Serious Games* (New York: Viking, 1970).

Castillo, Gloria A., *Left-Handed Teaching: Lessons in Affective Education* (New York: Praeger, 1974).

Gordon, Alice Kaplan, *Games for Growth: Educational Games in the Classroom* (Chicago: Science Research Associates, 1972).

Gorman, Alfred H., *Teachers and Learners: The Interactive Process of Education* (Boston: Allyn and Bacon, 1969).

Howard, Robert, *Human Psychology: Experiments in Awareness* (New York: Westinghouse Learning Corp., 1972).

_____, *Roles and Relationships: Exploring Attitudes and Values* (New York: Westinghouse Learning Corp., 1973).

James, Muriel, and Dorothy Jongeward, *Born to Win: Transactional Analysis with Gestalt Experiments* (Reading, Mass.: Addison-Wesley, 1971).

Miles, Matthew B., *Learning to Work in Groups* (New York: Teachers College Press, Columbia University, 1965).

Morgan, Richard, *Psychology: An Individualized Course* (Palo Alto, Calif.: Westinghouse Learning Press, 1970).

Pfeiffer, J. William, and John E. Jones, *A Handbook of Structured Experiences for Human Relations Training, Vol. I, II, III, IV* (Iowa City, Iowa: University Associates, 1969, 1970, 1971, 1974).

Reichert, Richard, *Self-Awareness Through Group Dynamics* (Dayton, Ohio: Pflaum/ Standard, 1970).

Reid, Avis, *Threads: Techniques for Human Relations Programs for Children.* (Glencoe, Minn.: Kopy Kat Printing, 1972).

Sax, Saville, and Sandra Hollander, *Reality Games* (New York: Macmillan, 1972).

Stanford, Gene, and Barbara Dodds Stanford, *Learning Discussion Skills Through Games* (New York: Citation, 1969).

Stanford, Gene, and Albert E. Roark, *Human Interaction in Education* (Boston: Allyn and Bacon, 1974).

Swell, Lila, *Educating for Success: Leaders' Guide* (Flushing, N.Y.: Queens College, 1972).

————, *Educating for Success: Workbook.* (Flushing, N.Y.: Queens College, 1972).

Taylor, John L., and Rex Walford, *Simulation in the Classroom* (Baltimore, Md.: Penguin Books, 1972).

Zuckerman, David W., and Robert E. Horn, *The Guide to Simulation Games for Education and Training* (Cambridge, Mass.: Information Resources, 1970).

B. HEALTH EDUCATION INSTRUCTIONAL STRATEGIES

As with the previous section of this bibliography, the following sources include learning experiences designed to require the active involvement of the learner. However, this section includes references to books which are specific to health education and will therefore require less by way of adaptation to the reader's instructional setting.

Boskins, Warren, and Michael Walsh, *Instructor's Guide to Essentials of Life and Health* (DelMar, Calif.: CRM Books, 1974).

Edwards, Gerald, *Reaching Out: The Prevention of Drug Abuse Through Increased Human Interaction* (New York: Holt, Rinehart & Winston, 1972).

Engs, Ruth, Eugene Barnes, and Molly Wantz, *Health Games Students Play* (Dubuque, Iowa: Kendall/Hunt, 1975).

Mayshark, Cyrus, and Roy A. Foster, *Methods in Health Education: A Workbook Using the Critical Incident Technique* (St. Louis: The C.V. Mosby Co., 1966).

Merki, Donald, and Bryan Gray, *Health Education Strategies* (Austin, Texas: Aus-Tex Duplicators, 1975).

Read, Donald A., and Walter H. Greene, *Creative Teaching in Health* (New York: Macmillan, 1971).

Samples, Bob, and Bob Wohlford, *Opening: A Primer for Self-Actualization* (Reading, Mass.: Addison-Wesley, 1973).

Savitz, Bobbie et al., *Go To Health* (New York: Dell, 1972).

Scott, Gwendolyn D., and Mona W. Carlo, *On Becoming A Health Educator* (Dubuque, Iowa: Wm. C. Brown Co., 1974).

Wood, G. Congdon (ed.), *Biology Experiments for High School Students* (New York: American Cancer Society, 1964).

C. HEALTH EDUCATION THEORY

The books referred to here provide rationales for the inclusion of health education in the school curriculum, descriptions of the school health program, conceptual frameworks for health education, and issues related to that subject area.

Fodor, John, and Gus Dalis, *Health Instruction: Theory and Application* (Philadelphia: Lea and Febiger, 1966).

Oberteuffer, Delbert, Orvis A. Harrelson, and Marion B. Pollock, *School Health Education* (5th ed.) (New York: Harper & Row, 1972).

Rathbone, Frank, and Estelle Rathbone, *Health and the Nature of Man* (New York: McGraw-Hill, 1971).

Read, Donald A., *New Directions in Health Education: Some Contemporary Issues for the Emerging Age* (New York: Macmillan, 1971).

Willgoose, Carl E., *Health Teaching in Secondary Schools* (Philadelphia: W. B. Saunders Co., 1972).

D. HEALTH SCIENCE CONTENT

For the health educator desiring more information about health content, the following sources are suggested. Among the content areas included in these books are drugs, family living, personal health, nutrition, safety, ecology, and community health.

Bruess, Clint E., and J. Thomas Fisher, *Selected Readings in Health* (Toronto: Macmillan, 1970).

CRM, *Life and Health* (2nd ed.) (New York: Random House, 1976).

Johnston, Lloyd, *Drugs and American Youth* (Ann Arbor, Mich.: Institute for Social Research, The University of Michigan, 1973).

Jones, Kenneth L., Louis W. Shainberg, and Curtis O. Byer, *Dimensions: A Changing Concept of Health* (San Francisco: Canfield Press, 1974).

LaPlace, John, *Health* (New York: Appleton-Century-Crofts, 1972).

Mayer, Jean, *Health* (New York: D. Van Nostrand, 1974).

Miller, Benjamin F., and John J. Burt, *Good Health: Personal and Community* (3rd ed.) (Philadelphia: W. B. Saunders Co., 1972).

Sinacore, John S., *Health: A Quality of Life* (2nd ed.) (New York: Macmillan, 1974).

E. HUMANISTIC EDUCATION

The reader interested in the educational philosophy espoused in this book, and interested in other expositions of this philosophy is directed to the following sources. These books present the humanistic educational philosophy, as well as suggestions regarding the actual implementation of this philosophy in school settings.

Borton, Terry, *Reach, Touch, and Teach: Students Concerns and Process Education* (New York: McGraw-Hill, 1970).

Kohl, Herbert, *The Open Classroom: A Practical Guide To A New Way of Teaching* (New York: Random House, 1969).

Rogers, Carl, *Freedom to Learn* (Columbus, Ohio: Charles E. Merrill, 1969).

Shumsky, Abraham, *In Search of Teaching Style* (New York: Appleton-Century-Crofts, 1968).

Swell, Lila, *Educating for Success: Theory Manual* (Flushing, N.Y.: Queens College, 1972).

Weinstein, Gerald, and Mario D. Fantini, (eds.), *Toward Humanistic Education: A Curriculum of Affect* (New York: Praeger, 1970).

F. VALUING

Since the valuing process is such an integral aspect of the mode of instruction suggested in this book, the following sources are cited for the reader interested in the theory upon which values clarification is based and other valuing activities.

Belina, Tom, *Values for Health* (Belmont, Calif.: Fearon, 1976).

Koberg, Don, and Jim Bagnall, *The Polytechnic School of Values: Values Tech* (Los Altos, Calif.: William Kaufman, 1976).

Morrison, Eleanor S., and Mila Underhill Price, *Values in Sexuality: A New Approach To Sex Education* (New York: Hart, 1974).

Osman, Jack Douglas, *The Feasibility of Using Selected Value Clarification Strategies in a Health Education Course for Future Teachers* (unpublished doctoral dissertation, The Ohio State University, 1971).

Raths, Louis E., Merrill Harmin, and Sidney B. Simon, *Values and Teaching: Working With Values in the Classroom* (Columbus, Ohio: Charles E. Merrill, 1966).

Simon, Sidney B., Leland W. Howe, and Howard Kirschenbaum, *Values Clarification: A Handbook of Practical Strategies for Teachers and Students* (New York: Hart, 1972).

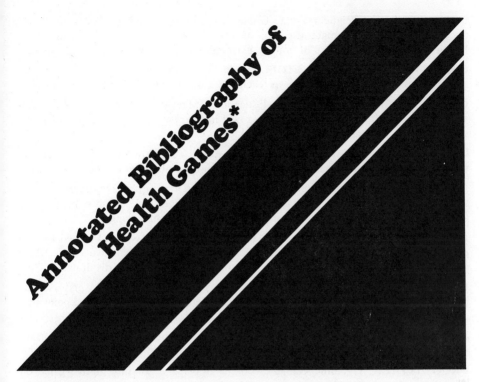

Annotated Bibliography of Health Games*

AGENDA, Educational Manpower, Inc., $15.00,† 18–39 players. A simulation of decision-making in a church assembly. Students assume roles of delegates and lobbyists in order to practice skills in negotiation, confrontation, political strategy, public speaking, and parliamentary procedure.

BODY TALK, Communication/Research/Machines, $8.00, 2–10 players. A game of nonverbal communication. Players attempt to express and receive emotions successfully without talking.

CAN OF SQUIRMS, Pennant Educational Materials, $5.95, 2 or more players. Encourages meaningful, interesting dialogue between individuals. Used as a discussion starter.

CHAOS, Lakeside, $4.39. CHAOS is used in health classes to illustrate confusion to the students. It is a game of memory and strategy. Discussion: What is chaos? Have you ever been confused? Does the noise bother you when you are trying to concentrate? How does it feel to be confused? Play the game twice, the first time with no noise, the second time with noise and confusion.

COMMUNITY LAND USE GAME, Educational Manpower, Inc., $75.00, 15–20 players. Teams possess money and buy land, construct buildings, and make investments. Can be used to explore issues related to environmental pollution.

---

* Some of these descriptions appeared in: Kenneth L. Packer, "Peer Training Through Game Utilization," *The Journal of School Health* **14,** 2, Feb. 1975, pp. 113–116. Copyright 1975 by the American School Health Association, Kent, Ohio 44240.

† Prices quoted were those in effect at time of writing.

COMPATIBILITY, Brigham Young University, 2 or more players. This game introduces considerations in mate selection such as: choice of mate, parental approval, length of courtship, maturity of couple, personality differences, and playing the field.

CORONARY CARE TIC-TAC-TOE, Spenco Medical Corp., $2.95, 2 players. This game utilizes graphics and humor to teach the nine known heart attack risk factors.

CRUEL CRUEL WORLD, Pennant Educational Materials, $8.95, 2–4 players. Develops an understanding of the values involved in the personal decisions as well as the values involved in that same person's goals.

CUTTING GRASS, Instructional Simulations, Inc., $35.00. Method for injecting peer-group pressure tactics and youth culture into drug abuse education programs.

DEELIE BOBBERS, Educational Manpower, Inc., $5.50, up to 24 players. A construction game to enhance understanding of group process and group dynamics and to aid players to develop imaginative approaches to problem-solving.

DISCUSSION, Pennant Educational Materials, $3.95, 2–5 players. Designed to help players understand that any event can offer both positive and negative values. Each player must cope with a situation using the positive and negative cards drawn.

DOWNER'S ROULETTE, Spenco Medical Corp., $49.50, 2 or more players. The game of chance that may save your life. This roulette wheel illustrates the point that downers should never be mixed.

DRINKING CLOCK, Spenco Medical Corp., $42.50, 2 or more players. The Drinking Clock teaches what you should know about drinking and driving.

DRUG ATTACK, Dynamic Games, $9.00, 3–5 players. An informative game on drug abuse that makes the student aware of how a community can deal with drug abuse, pushers, and users. The students must stop their attack, detect cause, and treat the victim.

THE END OF THE LINE, Educational Manpower, Inc., $75.00, 30–40 players. Intended to give participants a feel for what it is to grow old and what it is like to try to help people who are growing old.

ENERGY X, Educational Manpower, Inc., $19.50, entire class. A simulation game on natural resource allocation. Designed to provide an understanding of energy resource allocation, energy production, and other factors associated with the energy crisis.

FEELIN', Argus Communications, $8.50, 1–6 players. Helps players understand that their emotions are seldom simple. Players locate their feelings regarding various people and subjects by placing colorful wooden tokens in position on the game board.

GAMES PEOPLE PLAY, Masco, $12.50, 1–8 players. Game evolved from Eric Berne's book "Games People Play." Berne's theory of social interaction suggests the shifting of child–parent–adult role relationship give rise to games in which behavior and emotions of individuals are self-manipulated to gain societal approval.

GENERATION GAP, Western Publishing Co., $20.00, 4–10 players. This game simulates the interaction between an imaginary parent and son or daughter, with respect to five issues of disagreement (curfew, appearance, etc.) "Children" compete against "children" and "parents" against "parents" in attempting to develop the most satisfying relationship within the family. The game is highly flexible and can be adapted by users to the particular problems relevant to them.

GENERATION RAP, Educational Manpower, Inc., $10.00, 4–10 players. Opportunity to reverse parents' and children's roles and to see the other viewpoint.

GOMSTOM, Educational Manpower, Inc., $25.00, up to 40 players. The participants become the citizens of Gomstom—a typical community of the modern world with all the environmental problems of today.

GOOD-LOSER, Dietor, $12.00, 2–6 players. A weight control game for students.

HANG-UP, Synectics Education Systems, $16,00, 3–6 players. The setting is provided for the players to pantomime feelings, experienced in stress situations, to become aware of their real hang-ups, and to respond to the hang-ups of others.

HAPPINESS, Milton Bradley, $5.39, 2–6 players. The object of the game is to be the first player to reach the rainbow of happiness by filling a stand with the six required keys for happiness: Health, Faith, Love, Knowledge, Friendship, and Self Improvement. Discussion: Why do we need all the keys for happiness? Which do you feel is the most important?

HEADACHE, Kohner, $4.49, 2–4 players. This game can be used in health classes to illustrate reasons that so many people complain of headaches. The markers can represent people and the different types of trouble people run into. The leaders should make up problems that their students face daily.

INNOCENT UNTIL. . . , ABT Associates, Inc., $34.00, 13–32 players. Simulated courtroom drama. Players assume the roles of the people involved in a "drunk driving" case. Charge is manslaughter; the victim, a star high school athlete.

INSIGHT, Games Research, Inc., $15.00, 2–20 players. Players seek to gain insight by evaluating their own personalities and those of the other players. Personality perceptions are tested by comparing self-evaluation with evaluations made by other players.

JACK STRAWS, Parker Brothers, $1.99, 1 or more players. Similar to pick-up-sticks. The participants are to pick up the objects without touching another. The aim of the game is to develop manual dexterity and shows how an individual deals with frustration.

JIGSAW PUZZLES. Have groups of students put together puzzles to stimulate co-operation, or show lack of it, in the classroom. Any puzzle will do.

MAKE AND TAKE, ABT Associates, Inc., 2–50 players. Test takers and makers reverse roles, improve effectiveness in exams.

MATCH WITS, Pennant Educational Materials, $5.95, 2–40 players. Players are asked to identify the values involved in particular events. Helps players develop an understanding of the needs and the many values expressed in typical situations.

MY CUP RUNNETH OVER, Pennant Educational Materials, $7.95, 2–4 players. Helps players interpret the actions of other players, and practice recognizing their own verbal and nonverbal communications.

NEW TOWN, Educational Manpower, Inc., $28.00, 20 players. Bidding for land, erecting buildings, and holding town meetings simulates the requirements of modern town planning.

OPEN SPACE, Educational Manpower, Inc., $4.95, large group. A developer's proposal to build a huge shopping center stirs public debate. Representatives are from environmentalists, residents of slum neighborhood, parents favoring more recreation land, and local businessmen. A simulated public hearing is conducted.

PARENT–CHILD, Academic Games, Inc., $3.00, 4–10 players. This game simulates the interaction between an adolescent son or daughter and his or her parents, with respect to certain issues on which they have opposed attitudes.

PERSONALYSIS, Administrative Research Associates, 3 or 4 players. To see yourself as others see you. To aid the student in developing a deeper understanding of the strengths and weaknesses in personality.

POLLUTION, Educational Manpower, Inc., $24.00, 4–32 players. Four societal forces (business, citizens, conservationists, and state government) negotiate to develop a cleaner environment.

PROBLEM-SOLVING GAME, Didactic Systems, Inc., 16 players. The heart of the game is the nature of problem-solving and interpersonal relations.

RING TOSS GAME, Educational Manpower, Inc., $7.50, 1 or more players. A game used in achievement motivation training to help students analyze their own behavior and to help them explore risk-taking and the use of feedback.

SEARCH FOR MEANING, Pflaum/Standard Publishing Co., $33.95, 1–30 players. A tool kit of strategies and techniques which can help a person see more clearly the directions that person's day-to-day life choices are taking.

SEARCH FOR VALUES, Pflaum/Standard Publishing Co., $44.95, 1–30 players. Same idea as SEARCH FOR MEANING.

SIMULATION MULBERRY, Educational Manpower, Inc., $57.50, entire class. Students play the roles of citizens, city officials, and professional planners whose task it is to redevelop an area of 16 blocks in Mulberry.

SMOKERS ROULETTE, Spenco Medical Corp., $49.50, 2 or more players. Shows the diseases associated with smoking. The roulette wheel spins and selects diseases according to their probability of occurrence. Use poker chips for points.

SOUP'S ON, Dietor, $12.00, 2–40 players. A balanced diet bingo game. It teaches the composition of 84 common foods.

STAY ALIVE, Milton Bradley, $5.99. A game of survival testing strategies that will prevent the student from being eliminated. The students can also work in teams. Can be used to stimulate the following discussion: Have you ever come close to dying? How did you feel when you went down? Did you try to stay alive or hurt others? How did you feel when you made someone else go down?

TENSION, Kohner Brothers, $4.49, 2–4 players. This game is used in health classes to illustrate the feelings of tension. It is very important to define tension and exemplify feelings of tenseness. Discussion: What is tension? Have you ever felt tense? When? Has your mother or father ever been tense? How do you act, what do you do when you are tense?

THE SOCIAL SEMINAR, National Institute of Mental Health, $13.75, 32 players. This is a 2- to 5-hour game simulation of a community response to the problem of drug abuse. It is intended for use primarily by teachers, school personnel, and students interested in encouraging discussion on drug abuse prevention and education. Included are filmstrips, player's guide, role-playing activities.

THE UNGAME: TELL IT LIKE IT IS, Contemporary Design, $8.25, 3–6 players. The UNGAME has been described as "Transactional Analysis in a Box." This activity involves students in exploring their own feelings, attitudes, and motives, and to help them to become fully aware of their self-concepts. Game covers hopes, fears, joys, sorrows, philosophy, and ambitions.

TO DRINK OR NOT TO DRINK, Educational Manpower, Inc., $25.00, 5–16 players. Players are confronted with situations requiring drink or abstinence decisions, which must be made in the context of peer pressure.

THE TOTAL PERSON, Pennant Educational Materials, $10.00, small and large groups. Helps strengthen skills in decision-making, communication, self-awareness, interpersonal relations, and understanding human behavior.

TRIP OR TRAP BINGO, Spenco Medical Corp., $14.50, one or more players. Played just like regular bingo except that each bingo square shows a drug and a number. Game contains 40 bingo cards showing 75 different drugs.

TRIP OR TRAP PLAYING CARDS, Spenco Medical Corp., $3.95, one or more players. The numbered cards give detailed information and pictures of 36 different drugs and the face cards have slogans and humorous designs. You can play any card game with them.

TROUBLE, Kohner Brothers, Inc., $4.49, 2–4 players. This game is used in health classes to illustrate and discuss the ways and reasons students get into trouble. The teacher should make up a story involving students getting into trouble. Example: Chris broke a vase when her parents were at work. She then went to school. Her brother Tommy wants to tell on her, so he rushes home from school. She tries to get home before her parents and Tommy because she wants to clean up the broken vase. Have each marker represent a member of the family. Discuss: When do students get in trouble? How are they punished? Why do people misbehave? Why do people tell on each other?

VALUE BINGO, Pennant Educational Materials, $5.95, 2–40 players. Like bingo except caller reads statements instead of numbers and players identify the value category emphasized in the statement.

VALUES, Educational Manpower, Inc., $6.00, 3–6 players. Helps players determine what is important to them and why.

WHEELS, Dietor, $12.00, 2–40 players. A vitamin/mineral game. Covers 50 common foods.

WOMAN AND MAN, Educational Manpower, Inc., $8.00, 6 players. The war between the sexes, unlike most wars, has seen a lot of fraternizing across enemy lines. This is fortunate for love, babies, and unemployed poets; but it has also led to one sex trying to squelch the other. This game seeks to correct this problem by exploring the squelch process.

YOUTH CRISIS RESOLUTION GAME, Miller Productions Inc., $12.50, 3 or more players. This game was written to provide a value analysis, problem solving framework for dealing with such topics as student activism, drug use, and ecology. The games utilize a group process approach, role playing activities with debriefing, and follow-up materials.

YOUTH CULTURE GAME, Urbandyne, $15.00, 20 or more players. Role reversal and improvisational theater techniques provide a basis for communication between generations. Positive/negative aspects of both the current youthful subculture and the dominant mature American culture are presented.